Ageless Healing Through Nature

UNLOCK THE POWER OF NATURE TO HEAL, REJUVENATE, AND THRIVE AT ANY AGE

REENA AGARWAL

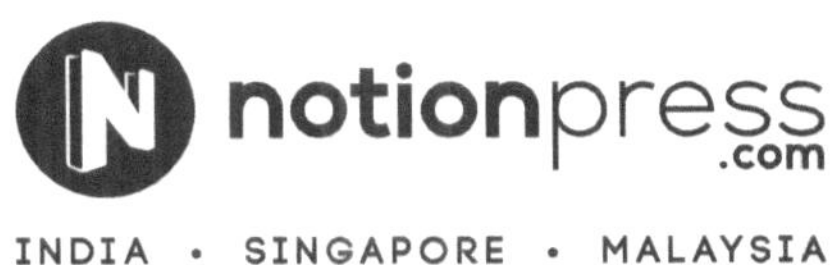

ISBN
Paperback 979-8-89906-939-0
Hardcase 979-8-89929-284-2

What if your body already knows how to heal itself?

This book is your invitation to rediscover the natural ways of healing—
without pills, without side effects. Through real-life inspiration, simple
routines, and ancient wisdom, you'll learn how to live pain-free, stress-
free, and disease-free—naturally.

If I could heal, so can you.

🌹 Dedication and 🍃 Acknowledgment

This book, *Ageless Healing Through Nature*, is a labor of love and a reflection of the journey that transformed my life. First and foremost, I bow in deep gratitude to the power of nature—its quiet wisdom, its gentle strength, and its ability to heal without asking for anything in return.

My heartfelt thanks to Dr. Biswaroop Roy Chowdhury, whose guidance illuminated my path to natural healing. Through his teachings and the principles of naturopathy, I was able to reclaim my health and free myself from years of medication. His work gave me the confidence to trust in nature and in my body's innate power to heal.

To my very precious family and loved ones—thank you for your unwavering support, patience, and encouragement during my healing journey. Your belief in me gave me the strength to keep going.

To every reader holding this book: You are the reason I wrote these pages. If my story can inspire even one person to take back control of their health and live a life of vitality, then this mission is fulfilled.

With deepest gratitude and healing light,

Reena Agarwal

Certified Nutrition & Wellness Coach

CONTENTS

- The body's incredible self-healing potential
- How nature heals on physical, emotional, and spiritual levels
- The three pillars: Nourishment, Movement, and Mindset
- Breaking free from medication dependency
- ❧ My journey: Healing high blood pressure through nature

- The healing power of whole, plant-rich foods
- Anti-inflammatory and disease-fighting superfoods
- Natural detox through raw foods, juices, nuts, and seeds
- Building your personalized healing diet
- ❧ My healing transformation through food

- The importance of daily movement for longevity
- Yoga, stretching, and functional movement for vitality
- Deep breathing and pranayama for stress relief
- Simple practices for pain and stiffness relief
- ❧ My daily barefoot walks, yoga, and hot water therapy

❧ PREFACE

"When we return to nature, we return to ourselves. Healing begins the moment we choose to nourish, not neglect."

— Reena Agarwal

Ageless Healing Through Nature is more than a guide—it's a return to the wisdom of our roots. In today's world, where stress, fatigue, and disease are all too common, we have forgotten that our bodies are innately designed to heal. Nature offers us everything we need to rejuvenate.

As a Certified Nutrition and Wellness Coach, I've worked intensively with natural healing and have personally experienced the miracle of reversing chronic illness—without medicines—by using nature as my healer. In this book, I am sharing my most valuable personal experiences and insights with you, the reader, in the hope that they will inspire and empower your own healing journey.

You'll discover how simple yet powerful practices can transform your life at any age. This is a journey to awaken your body's intelligence and rediscover the joy of living fully, naturally, and consciously.

Whether you're dealing with illness, feeling disconnected from your body, or simply curious about living a healthier life, this book is an invitation to heal—gently and holistically—with the help of nature.

Let this be your starting point to thrive—not just survive

– Reena Agarwal

❧ ABOUT THE AUTHOR

Reena Agarwal is a passionate **Nutrition and Wellness Coach** dedicated to empowering individuals to reclaim their health naturally. With a deep-rooted belief in **naturopathy and holistic healing,** she has spent years guiding people toward a **medicine-free lifestyle** by harnessing the power of nature.

Through her extensive work in **natural healing, nutrition, and wellness,** Reena has helped countless individuals overcome chronic health challenges, reduce stress, and achieve a state of vibrant well-being. She specializes in **plant-based nutrition, detoxification, and mind-body healing techniques,** proving that true wellness is within reach for everyone at any age.

Her approach is simple yet profound: **nourish the body, move with purpose, and cultivate a healing mindset.** By blending **scientific insights** with **time-honored natural remedies,** she empowers her readers and clients to break free from dependency on medication and embrace a **life of vitality, balance, and joy.**

With this book, Reena hopes to inspire you to **trust in the healing power of nature** and embark on a journey toward **lifelong health and rejuvenation.**

Reena Agarwal: A passionate Nutrition & Wellness Coach and advocate for natural wellness

> "True healing begins when we stop fighting symptoms and start listening to our bodies. Nature holds every answer—if I could heal through its gifts, so can you."

– Reena Agarwal
Certified Nutrition and Wellness Coach

REVIEWS FROM OTHERS

❉ Praise for Ageless Healing Through Nature:

"This book is a breath of fresh air in a world full of pills and prescriptions. Reena's journey is not only inspiring—it's a wake-up call. Her practical, nature-based approach gave me hope and helped me take my first step toward true healing."

– Meera S., Holistic Wellness Practitioner

"Reading this book felt like a warm conversation with a wise friend. Simple, sincere, and incredibly empowering—Ageless Healing Through Nature is the guide I didn't know I needed."

– Anita R., Reader & Wellness Enthusiast

"A must-read for anyone tired of being dependent on medications. Reena Agarwal beautifully captures the essence of healing with nature—her personal journey alone is worth the read!"

– Dr. Kavita Mehra, Integrative Medicine Specialist

"This book is a healing gift. Reena's practical steps, rooted in nature and ancient wisdom, bring hope, energy, and clarity to the health journey."

– Rajiv Sharma, Certified Yoga Therapist

"Reena Agarwal shows us that the path to vibrant health isn't complicated—it's natural. Her story is moving, her guidance is grounded, and her wisdom is empowering."

– Anjali Verma, Holistic Nutritionist

THE POWER OF NATURAL HEALING

In a world where hospitals are full, prescriptions are overflowing, and stress has become a silent epidemic, many of us are quietly asking: **Is this how life is meant to be?**

Every day, more people wake up tired, overwhelmed, and dependent on medications just to get through the day. Chronic diseases like high blood pressure, diabetes, anxiety, and fatigue have become so common that we've accepted them as "normal." But the truth is — **being unwell is not your destiny.** There is a better way. A gentler, deeper, more sustainable path.

🚨 The Modern Health Crisis

We live in an era of technological advancements and modern medicine, yet people are sicker than ever. We're plugged in, but deeply disconnected — from our bodies, our food, our emotions, and from nature itself. Fast food, quick fixes, and an "always-on" lifestyle are costing us not just our health, but our joy, vitality, and peace of mind.

💊 The Limitations of Conventional Medicine

Conventional medicine has undoubtedly saved lives and plays a critical role in acute care. But when it comes to chronic disease, it often focuses on managing symptoms rather than healing the root cause. It's a system of control, not liberation — and it can leave people feeling stuck, helpless, and dependent.

🌿 Nature: The Original Healer

Everything your body needs to heal, thrive, and glow with vitality is found in nature. The fresh foods that nourish your cells, the herbs that gently detoxify your body, the sunlight that boosts your immunity, the soil beneath your feet that rebalances your energy — it's all there, waiting to support you. **Healing is not outside of you; it's already within you. You** simply need to reconnect.

Nature doesn't rush. It doesn't overwhelm. It nurtures, balances, and restores — gently but powerfully.

📖 What You Can Expect from This Book

Ageless Healing Through Nature is not just a book — it's a guide, a companion, and an invitation to return to your most natural, vibrant self.

You'll also read my personal healing journey — from a life of medication and fatigue to one of freedom, energy, and joy. My hope is that **my story lights a spark in you** — to believe that healing is possible, and that you are more powerful than you've been led to believe.

🌸 **"Healing is not something you chase. It's something you allow, through alignment with the rhythms of nature."**

Are you ready to begin? Let's walk this path together — back to nature, back to health, and back to you. 🌿

THE FOUNDATION OF NATURAL HEALING

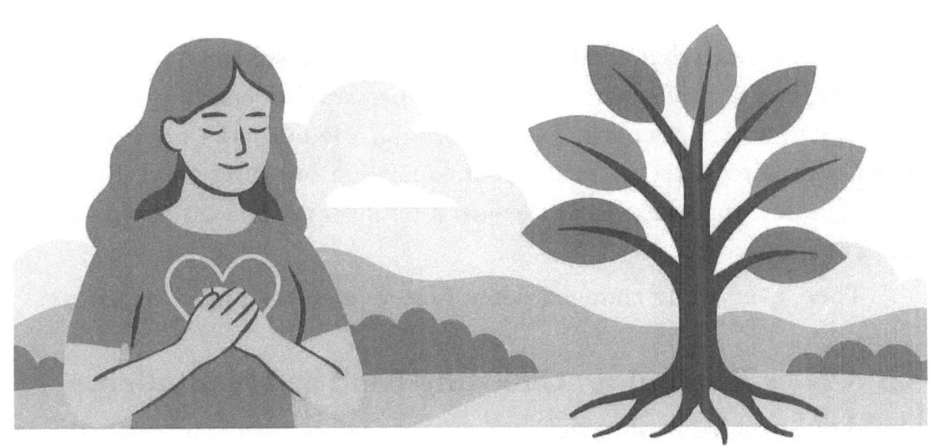

Understanding the body's self-healing abllities

How nature supports healing at every level--physical, emotional, and spiritual

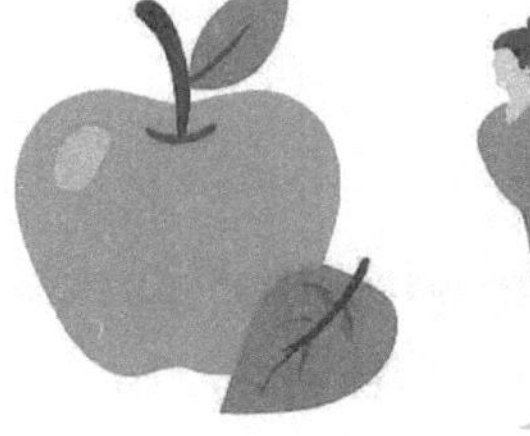 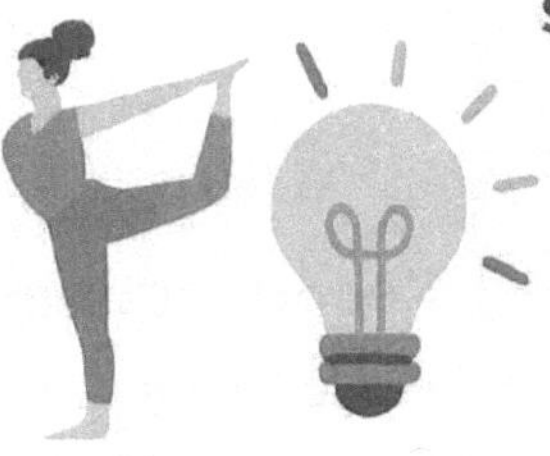 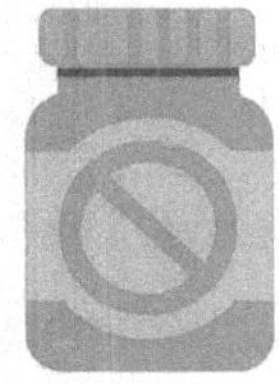

The three pillars of health: Nourishment, and movement, and mindset

Breaking free from the dependency on medication

This chapter lays the groundwork for the reader's journey toward **ageless healing through nature**, focusing on **the body's innate ability to heal, how nature supports holistic wellness, and how to move beyond dependence on medication.**

"Nature is a Miraculous Healing Balm." — Lori Deschene

❧ My Journey: Healing Through Nature

There was a time when I believed that medication was my only hope. For **five long years**, I lived with **high blood pressure**, depending on pills to keep my numbers in check. Every morning, I would take my prescribed dose, hoping to keep my health from spiraling out of control. But deep inside, I knew this wasn't a cure—just a temporary fix. I often wondered, *Is there another way?*

Then, everything changed when I discovered the **power of nature.**

🍎 A New Beginning: Choosing Food as My Medicine

One day, I decided to stop fighting against my body and start **nourishing it instead.** I made a radical shift—**no more processed food, no dairy products, no refined sugar, and no packaged products.** Instead, I turned to nature's purest gifts:

The more I embraced whole, living foods, the more I felt my **body waking up,** as if it had been craving this nourishment all along.

👣 Walking Barefoot: Reconnecting with the Earth

Alongside my dietary shift, I made a commitment to **spend time in nature daily.** Every morning, I would step out into the garden, remove my shoes, and **walk barefoot on the cool, dewy grass.**

This practice, known as **earthing,** had a profound impact on my well-being. I could **feel the energy of the Earth flow into me,** dissolving stress, calming my mind, and balancing my body. Science confirms that **walking barefoot** reduces inflammation, improves circulation, and stabilizes the nervous system. I didn't just feel the difference—I **became the difference.**

🧘 Yoga & Breathwork: Healing Through Movement

I also introduced **daily yoga and stretching** into my routine, even if just for 20-30 minutes. With each stretch and deep breath, I could feel the **stiffness and tension melting away.**

But what truly transformed me was **pranayama**—the art of breath control. Every day, I practiced deep, conscious breathing, allowing oxygen to **flood my cells, energize my brain, and cleanse my body from within.**

- **Deep belly breathing** lowered my stress
- **Alternate nostril breathing** balanced my energy
- **Slow exhalations** calmed my racing thoughts

With each breath, I felt **lighter, stronger, and more alive.**

🧘🔯 The Power of a Stress-Free Mindset

One of the biggest lessons I learned on my healing journey was that **stress is the silent killer.** No matter how well you eat, no matter how much you exercise, if your mind is filled with stress, **your body will suffer.**

So, I made a choice: **I refused to let stress control my life.**

- ☑ I started meditating every day, even if just for a few minutes.
- ☑ I practiced gratitude—focusing on what was going right instead of what was wrong.
- ☑ I embraced **joy, laughter, and simplicity,** letting go of things I couldn't control.

Slowly but surely, I felt **my heart rate stabilize, my blood pressure normalize, and my body thrive without medication.**

✿ Breaking Free: A Life Without Pills

Months into this new lifestyle, I felt a **dramatic shift.** My energy soared, my mood improved, and when I checked my blood pressure—it was **perfectly normal.** My doctor was astonished. I had done what seemed impossible—I had healed myself **without a single pill.**

Today, I live a **vibrant, medication-free life,** and I feel better than ever. I share my journey because I want **you** to know that this is possible for you too. **Your body is designed to heal—when you give it what it truly needs.**

✿   You don't need more medicine—you need more nature.

✿   You don't need suppression—you need transformation.

✿   You don't need to fight your body—you need to nourish it.

Are you ready to take the first step toward **ageless healing?** 🌱 ✦

1. ☽ Understanding the Body's Self-Healing Abilities

Your body is not just a machine—it is a living, breathing, adapting organism equipped with the wisdom to heal itself. Every second, your cells are regenerating, detoxifying, and defending you from harm.

Cuts close, bones mend, and fevers fight off infections—this is the magic of your built-in healing system. But when we overload the body with processed foods, stress, pollution, and synthetic chemicals, we interfere with this natural process. Healing isn't something that always requires external intervention—it's a matter of **removing the blocks and supplying the body with the right tools.**

🌱 *"Health is not something you acquire—it is something you align with."*

◇ **Key Points:**

- The human body is designed to **heal itself** when given the right environment and support.

- The **immune system, microbiome, and nervous system** play crucial roles in self-repair.

- The body constantly **regenerates:**
  - Skin renews every **27 days**
  - The liver can **regrow itself** even if 70% is removed
  - The gut lining **regenerates** every **2-5 days**

◇ **Examples & Interesting Facts:**

- **Wound Healing:** When you get a cut, your body **automatically triggers clotting, inflammation, and new cell growth** without intervention.

- **Placebo Effect:** Studies show that the mind alone can stimulate healing, proving the power of belief in recovery.

- The human body is a **miraculous self-healing machine**—it constantly repairs, regenerates, and restores balance without any external intervention.

- When you cut your finger, **does it heal on its own? Yes!** That's your body's natural intelligence at work. Imagine if we could harness that same power for chronic diseases.

- The problem? We often overload our bodies with **processed foods, stress, toxins, and medications,** which block this **self-repair mechanism.**

- When we remove the obstacles and provide **natural, nourishing support,** healing becomes effortless.

🔖 **Example:** Many chronic diseases like high blood pressure, diabetes, and digestive issues improve significantly—or even disappear—when people switch to a whole-food, plant-based diet.

◇ **Actionable Tip for Readers:**

Start **trusting your body** by reducing unnecessary medications and relying on natural healing first when possible.

2. How Nature Supports Healing at Every Level— Physical, Emotional, and Spiritual

Nature isn't just a backdrop to our lives; it's an essential partner in healing. It provides us with **food, fresh air, sunlight, and grounding energy** to support all levels of health.

Nature is the original healer. It nourishes not only the body, but also the mind and soul. Here's how:

◇ **Key Points:**

🦴 **Physical Healing:**

- **Sunlight** boosts vitamin D, strengthens immunity, and supports hormonal health.(Explained in detail in chapter 7)
- **Fresh air** oxygenates your blood, calms the nervous system, and improves mental clarity.
- **Walking barefoot (earthing)** reduces inflammation and enhances sleep.(Explained in detail in chapter 7)
- **Whole, plant-based foods** detoxify, rejuvenate cells, and fuel regeneration.
- **Water** detoxifies the body and improves cellular function

💙 **Emotional Healing:**

- Nature soothes anxiety and uplifts your mood.
- Listening to birdsong, feeling the breeze, or tending a garden fosters joy and inner peace.
- Practices like **forest bathing** (shinrin-yoku in Japan) have been scientifically shown to lower cortisol and reduce depression.
- Exposure to nature **reduces stress, anxiety, and depression—** scientific studies prove that spending time in green spaces **lowers cortisol** (stress hormone) levels.
- Natural environments **activate the parasympathetic nervous system,** shifting us into a state of **relaxation and repair.**

🧠 Spiritual Healing:

- Nature connects you to something greater than yourself.
- Time in natural environments invites mindfulness, gratitude, and a sense of purpose.
- Stillness in nature quiets mental noise and **reconnects you to your intuitive wisdom.**
- Being in nature fosters **inner peace, mindfulness, and a deep connection with the universe.**
- Ancient wisdom traditions and modern research both confirm that time spent in nature **enhances mental clarity and emotional resilience.**

🌿 *"In every walk with nature, one receives far more than he seeks."* – *John Muir*

📌 **Example:** Have you ever noticed how a walk in the park can instantly uplift your mood? That's nature healing you—**physically, emotionally, and spiritually.**

◇ **Interesting Facts:**

- **Forest Bathing in Japan:** The practice of "Shinrin-Yoku" (forest bathing) has been scientifically proven to **boost immunity and lower stress hormones.**
- **Sunlight and Healing:** Exposure to **morning sunlight** (without sunscreen for 10-15 minutes) helps regulate **circadian rhythms, improve sleep, and increase vitamin D production.**

◇ **Actionable Tip for Readers:**

Spend at least **20 minutes daily in nature** to experience its healing benefits.

3. △ The Three Pillars of Health: Nourishment, Movement, and Mindset

To create lasting wellness, you need a strong foundation built on these three interconnected elements:

i). Nourishment: Food as Medicine. (Details are discussed in chapter 2)

- Choose vibrant, living foods: **fresh fruits, vegetables, green juices, soaked nuts, seeds, sprouts, coconut water.**
- Eliminate what the body doesn't recognize: **animal products, dairy products, processed and packaged foods.**
- Food can either be the slowest form of poison or the most **powerful medicine.**

> "Let food be thy medicine and medicine be thy food."
>
> – Hippocrates

◇ **Key Points:**

☑ **Whole vs. Processed Foods** – Processed foods strip away nutrients and introduce harmful additives that burden the body, while whole foods provide vitamins, minerals, and enzymes needed for healing.

☑ **Eat the Rainbow** – Different colors in fruits and vegetables represent unique healing properties. For example, leafy greens detoxify, berries protect cells, and oranges boost immunity.

☑ **Seasonal & Local Eating** – Consuming foods that grow naturally in your environment enhances digestion and strengthens immunity.

Nature provides **everything we need** to heal through food—herbs, fruits, vegetables, seeds, and nuts.

◇ **Interesting Fact:**

The gut produces **95% of serotonin,** meaning diet affects not just digestion but **mood and mental health** too.

◇ **Actionable Tip for Readers:**

Drink **lemon water every morning** to support digestion and detoxification.

ii). **Movement: The Key to Lifelong Vitality.** (Details are discussed in chapter 3)

- Daily movement stimulates **circulation, oxygenates tissues, and supports detox.**
- **Walking barefoot, gentle yoga, stretching, and functional exercises** moves stagnant energy and keep you youthful.
- **Movement** is medicine—it strengthens not just the body, but also the mind and spirit.

◇ **Key Points:**

- **Sitting is the new smoking** – lack of movement contributes to disease.
- Gentle movements like **yoga, stretching, and walking** improve circulation, reduce stress, and ease pain.
- The **lymphatic system** (which removes toxins) has no pump—it depends on movement.

◇ **Interesting Fact:**

Just **30 minutes of walking daily** can reduce the risk of chronic disease by **40%**.

◇ **Actionable Tip for Readers:**

Try **5-minute deep breathing and stretching** every morning to wake up your body.

iii). **Mindset: The Healing Power of Thoughts.** (Details are discussed in chapter 4)

- Your thoughts shape your biology. **Chronic stress or negativity** suppresses immunity and delays healing.
- **Mindfulness, meditation, gratitude, and emotional resilience** are just as vital as diet and exercise.
- When you believe in your body's **ability to heal,** you unlock its full potential.

◇ **Key Points:**

- Chronic stress **weakens immunity** and **increases inflammation.**
- **Gratitude and positive thinking** trigger brain chemistry that supports healing.
- Meditation, affirmations, and deep breathing reduce **cortisol and improve cellular health.**

◇ **Interesting Fact:**

Studies show **daily gratitude practices** can lower inflammation markers and **reduce heart disease risk.**

✎ **Example:** Scientific studies show that people with a **positive outlook and a strong belief in healing** recover faster from illness.

◇ **Actionable Tip for Readers:**

- Write down **3 things you're grateful for** every morning to shift into a healing mindset.

🧠 "True healing begins with the belief that you can heal."

4. 🔓 Breaking Free from the Dependency on Medication

In today's fast-paced world, we often reach for **quick fixes**—especially when it comes to our health. **Popping a pill** has become the new norm for everything from **headaches to high blood pressure, anxiety to indigestion.** But what if true healing doesn't lie in suppressing symptoms, but in addressing the **root cause?**

❂ Reena's Journey: From Pills to Power

I personally lived with high blood pressure for over five years, reliant on daily medication. I believed it was something I would manage for life. But everything changed when I shifted my focus to **food as medicine.** By embracing a healing lifestyle—filled with raw fruits, vegetable juices, soaked nuts and seeds, and mindful practices like walking barefoot, yoga, and stress reduction—I not only improved my health but **completely eliminated my need for medication.** Today, I am free of **high blood pressure** and full of energy, clarity, and peace.

☑ The Reality of Medication Dependence

Many people live their lives dependent on medications for years, sometimes decades, believing they have no other choice. While modern medicine has its place—especially in emergencies and acute conditions—long-term reliance on drugs can often mask the **real issues and create side effects** that require even more medication. It becomes a cycle that's hard to break.

🌱 A New Perspective on Healing

Breaking free from this cycle doesn't mean rejecting medicine entirely—it means **reclaiming the power to support your body's natural healing process.** Your body is a miraculous, self-healing organism. When given the right environment—nourishing foods, movement, clean air, rest, and a calm mind—it knows how to repair, regenerate, and thrive.

💡 What You Can Do:

- **Start small:** Replace one processed meal a day with a raw plant-based meal.
- **Hydrate wisely:** Water is nature's cleanser—sip throughout the day.
- **Move mindfully:** Daily walks, gentle yoga, or stretching help release toxins and stimulate healing.
- **Breathe deeply:** A few minutes of focused breathing calms the nervous system and supports detox.
- **Question the root:** For every medication, ask: *What is the real cause of this symptom?*

⬚ Medication Reduction: Always With Caution

Breaking free doesn't mean quitting all meds overnight. It's a **gradual journey** that should be done mindfully and, ideally, with the guidance of a trusted wellness expert or integrative physician. As your body strengthens and your health improves through natural methods, medications often become less necessary.

❀ **"You were not born to live on pills. You were born to heal."**

The modern world often treats **symptoms** instead of causes. We've come to rely heavily on medications that:

- **Suppress** natural signals from the body.
- Cause long-term **side effects** and **dependency**.
- Mask the **root issues** without addressing them.

Instead, natural healing **empowers you** to:

- Take **responsibility** for your health.
- **Learn** what your body truly needs.
- **Reduce** or **eliminate** medications safely with lifestyle shifts (under proper guidance).

◇ **Key Points:**

- Medications **often treat symptoms,** not root causes.
- **Overuse of antibiotics** can harm the gut microbiome, weakening immunity.
- Many chronic diseases (diabetes, hypertension) are **lifestyle-related** and can be reversed naturally.
- The goal is not to reject medicine but to **empower yourself** so that you don't need it.

How to break free?

☑ **Remove triggers** (processed food, toxins, stress)

☑ **Support healing naturally** (nutrition, movement, mindset)

☑ **Listen to your body**—it always signals what it needs

◇ **Examples & Interesting Facts:**

- The **opioid crisis** started because people were overprescribed painkillers instead of being taught natural pain relief methods.

- Studies show **lifestyle changes** can reverse **type 2 diabetes** and even some heart diseases.

◇ **Actionable Tip for Readers:**

- Before reaching for medicine, ask: **"Can I solve this naturally first?"**

Conclusion of the Chapter

☑ Summarize the key ideas:

- Your body is built to **heal itself** when given the right conditions.

- Nature is the best **doctor**—providing food, movement, and mental balance.

- Relying less on medication starts with **understanding the root cause** of issues and addressing them naturally.

◇ **Final Takeaway for Readers:**

Commit to ONE small change today—more natural foods, daily movement, or stress reduction—**and feel the difference.**

Chapter 2

NUTRITION AS MEDICINE

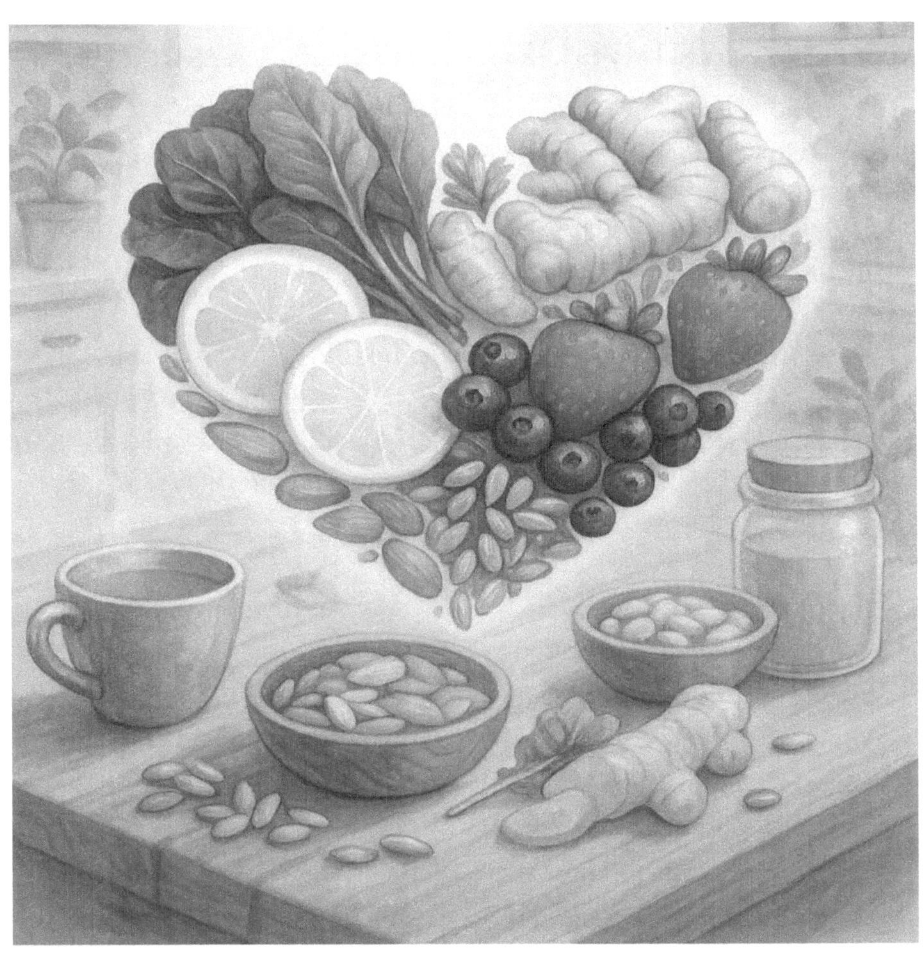

This chapter will explore how **whole foods can heal the body**, reduce inflammation, prevent disease, and boost longevity. It will also guide readers on how to create a **plant-rich healing diet** that promotes vitality.

Food is not just fuel; it is the foundation of our health. Every bite we take has the potential to heal or harm. When we embrace whole, natural foods, we allow our bodies to regenerate, detoxify, and thrive without the crutch of medications.

"Diet is essential key to all successful healing".- Joseph Raynauld Ramond 🖉

Personal Story: *I was dependent on high blood pressure medication for five years until I embraced nature's healing power. By changing my diet and lifestyle, I completely reversed my condition and freed myself from medication. If I could do it, you can too!*

1. The Healing Power of Whole Foods

Nature has provided us with everything we need to nourish and heal ourselves. Whole foods—foods in their natural, unprocessed state—are rich in essential nutrients, fiber, antioxidants, and enzymes that support every system of the body.

◇ **Key Points:**

☑ **Whole Foods vs. Processed Foods:**

- Processed and packaged foods contribute to **inflammation, disrupt digestion, and weaken the immune system.**
- Whole, plant-based foods provide essential **vitamins, minerals, antioxidants, and fiber to heal the body naturally.**

☑ **A Healing, Anti-Inflammatory Diet:**

- Prioritize **fresh, natural foods** that support cellular repair and longevity.
- Incorporate **fruits, soaked dry fruits, soaked seeds, sprouts, coconut, and fresh juices** to nourish the body.
- Avoid **refined sugars, processed oils, artificial additives, and preservatives** that lead to chronic illness.

☑ **Healing Superfoods:**

- **Fresh Turmeric & Ginger** – Powerful anti-inflammatory and immune-boosting spices.

- **Garlic** – Natural antibiotic, supports heart health and fights infections.

- **Leafy Greens (Spinach, Kale, Moringa,Pan leaves etc.)** – Rich in chlorophyll, detoxifies and provides essential micronutrients.

- **Soaked Nuts & Seeds (Almonds, Walnuts, Cashews, Raisins, Figs, Dates, Flax seeds, Chia seeds, Sunflower Seeds, Pumpkin Seeds)** – Loaded with healthy fats, protein, and brain-supporting nutrients.

- **Coconut Water, Coconut Flesh, Coconut Oil** – Hydrates, supports digestion, and provides quick energy.

- **Fermented Foods (Homemade Probiotic Drinks like Kanji, Pickled Vegetables)** – Promote gut health and improve nutrient absorption.

- **Fresh Juices (Vegetable & Fruit Juices Without Sugar, Salt or Preservatives)** – Provide natural enzymes, vitamins, and hydration for cell repair.

☑ **The Power of Simplicity in Eating:**

- Focus on **raw, whole, plant-based foods** for maximum nutrition.

- Eat **seasonal, local produce** for better nutrient absorption and balance.

- **Hydration is key**—start the day with warm water, herbal teas, or fresh coconut water.

Nature provides **everything we need** to heal through food—herbs, fruits, vegetables, seeds, and nuts.

🔑 **Example:** Instead of reaching for refined cereal in the morning, a vibrant fruit bowl with soaked nuts and seeds supplies energy, fiber, and essential fatty acids for a strong start to the day.

◇ **Examples & Interesting Facts:**

- **Blue Zones Diets:** The longest-living people in the world (Okinawa, Sardinia, etc.) eat **mostly whole plant-based foods** with little processed food.

- **The Hippocrates Quote:** "Let food be thy medicine and medicine be thy food" is now supported by **modern nutritional science.**

◇ **Actionable Tip for Readers:**

- **Choose whole over processed** – Eat foods in their **most natural state** (e.g., fresh apples instead of apple juice).

2. Anti-Inflammatory and Disease-Fighting Superfoods

Inflammation is the root cause of most chronic diseases, from arthritis to heart disease. The good news? Certain foods have natural anti-inflammatory properties, helping to reduce pain, swelling, and cellular damage.

🍃 **Top Anti-Inflammatory Superfoods:**

- **Fresh Turmeric & Ginger** – Nature's most powerful anti-inflammatory duo, reducing pain and promoting healing.

- **Berries (Blueberries, Acai, Goji)** – Rich in antioxidants that protect against oxidative stress, premature aging and disease.

- **Dark Leafy Greens** – Kale, spinach, pan and moringa leaves are packed with vitamins, minerals and chlorophyll, which detoxifies and purifies the blood.

- **Coconut & Avocado** – Provide healthy fats that support brain function and reduce inflammation.

- **Nuts & Seeds (Soaked)** – Almonds, walnuts, flaxseeds, and chia seeds deliver essential Omega-3s and minerals.

- **Garlic & Onions** – Contain sulfur compounds that boost immunity and fight infections.

🔖 **Example:** A golden turmeric milk (made with coconut milk, fresh turmeric and black pepper) can work wonders in **reducing joint pain and strengthening immunity.**

◇ **Key Points:**

- Chronic inflammation is the **root cause of many diseases** (arthritis, heart disease, diabetes, cancer).

- **Anti-inflammatory superfoods** can reduce pain, heal the gut, and prevent disease.

- Foods rich in **antioxidants, polyphenols, and healthy fats** fight cellular damage.

◇ **Interesting Facts:**

- Fresh Turmeric's active compound (**Curcumin**) is scientifically proven to be as effective as some anti-inflammatory drugs.

- **A handful of soaked walnuts daily** can reduce the risk of heart disease by 30%.

◇ **Actionable Tip for Readers:**

- Start the day with a **healing smoothie** packed with **berries, greens, and fresh turmeric.**(no milk or dairy products)

3. Detoxifying the Body Naturally with Food

Our bodies accumulate toxins daily—from the air we breathe, the water we drink, and the food we eat. Natural detoxification through food helps cleanse our system, boosting energy, digestion, and mental clarity.

💧 Natural Detox Foods & Practices:

- **Hydration is Key** – Start the day with **warm lemon water** to flush out toxins.

- **Fasting & Light Eating** – Giving the digestive system a break with fruit-based breakfasts or **intermittent fasting** can help eliminate waste.

- **Raw & Fermented Foods** – Cabbage, kimchi, and coconut yogurt feed gut-friendly bacteria, essential for digestion.

- **Herbal Infusions** – Tulsi, dandelion, and mint teas support liver detox and improve metabolism.

✎ **Example:** Replacing coffee with fresh green juice (celery, cucumber, lemon, ginger) can rejuvenate your body and mind.

◇ **Key Points:**

- The body naturally detoxifies through the **liver, kidneys, and lymphatic system.**
- Processed foods, chemicals, and toxins slow down detoxification.
- Eating **detoxifying foods** helps the body flush out toxins naturally.

◇ **Best Detox Foods:**

- ✔ **Lemon & Warm Water** – Kickstarts digestion and flushes toxins in the morning.
- ✔ **Beets & Carrots** – Support liver detox and improve bile flow.
- ✔ **Cruciferous Vegetables (Broccoli, Cauliflower, Cabbage)** – Help neutralize harmful toxins.
- ✔ **Cilantro & Parsley** – Aid in heavy mental detox.
- ✔ **Fresh Green leaves Tea & Herbal Teas** – Provide antioxidants and support liver function.

◇ **Interesting Facts:**

1. **The Liver's Superpower**
   The liver is the only internal organ that can **completely regenerate itself.** Even after significant damage or surgical removal of part of it, the liver can regrow if provided with the **right nutrients** and a break from toxins. This is why nutrient-dense foods and natural detox practices are crucial in your healing journey.

2. **Fasting Boosts Natural Healing**
   Practicing **intermittent fasting**—such as fasting for **12–16 hours** daily—gives the digestive system a break and activates the body's **autophagy process,** where it clears out damaged cells and toxins. This can **boost immunity, reduce inflammation,** and enhance overall vitality.

3. **The Kidneys: Silent Guardians of Health**
    Your kidneys work tirelessly to **filter over 50 gallons of blood** daily, removing waste and balancing fluids and minerals. They are essential for detoxification and blood pressure regulation. Drinking enough water, eating **potassium-rich foods** like bananas and sweet potatoes, and reducing salt and processed foods can **protect and support kidney function** naturally.

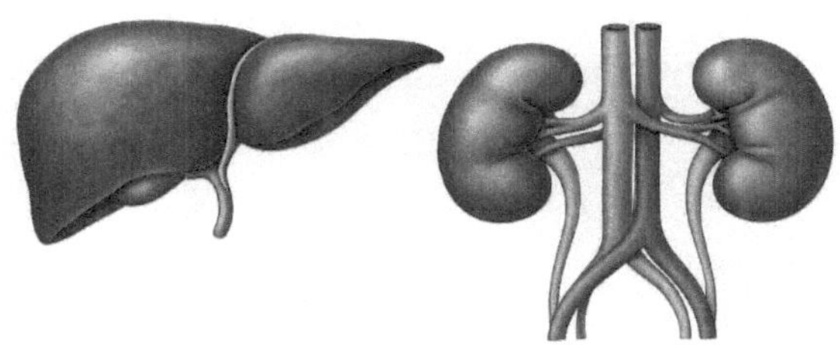

❈ The Liver: A Remarkable Organ of Regeneration

The **liver** is one of the most powerful and resilient organs in the human body. What makes it truly extraordinary is its **ability to regenerate—even after up to 70% of it has been damaged or removed**, the liver can grow back to its full size and function, *if* it is supported properly.

◇ **How the Liver Heals:**

When given the **right nutrients** and a break from toxins, the liver begins its natural repair process. Healing foods like:

- **Leafy greens**
- **Beetroot**
- **Fresh Turmeric**
- **Fresh fruits (especially citrus and berries)**
- **Cruciferous vegetables (like broccoli and cabbage)**
- **Plenty of water and herbal teas**
- … all help flush out toxins, reduce inflammation, and boost regeneration.

⬣ **Avoiding harmful inputs like:**

- Processed foods
- Alcohol
- Excess medications
- Sugar and fried foods
- … is equally important to allow your liver to heal.

This fact beautifully illustrates the body's **innate wisdom and power to heal itself**—a core message in this book *"Ageless Healing Through Nature."*

Intermittent Fasting (IF)

❋ **Intermittent Fasting (IF):** is an eating pattern that cycles between periods of eating and fasting. It doesn't focus on *what* you eat, but *when* you eat.

◇ **Brief Overview:**
- **Popular methods** include:
  - **16/8 method:** Fast for 16 hours, eat within an 8-hour window (e.g., eating between 10 AM – 6 PM).
  - **5:2 method:** Eat normally for 5 days, and restrict calories (500–600) on 2 non-consecutive days.
  - **24-hour fast:** Fasting for a full day once a week or once in 15 days with only coconut water within an 8-hour eating window (e.g., 10 AM – 6 PM) and normal water.

◇ **Health Benefits:**
- Helps in **weight loss** and **fat burning**
- Improves **insulin sensitivity** and blood sugar control
- Supports **cellular repair** and **autophagy** (body's natural detox and repair process)
- May reduce **inflammation** and boost **mental clarity**
- Supports **longevity** and **disease prevention**

◇ **Important Note:**

It's not suitable for everyone—especially those with certain health conditions or pregnant women—so it's good to consult a healthcare provider before starting.

❈ Reviving Kidney Health Naturally

Contrary to popular belief, **damaged kidneys can begin to heal**—especially in the early stages—when supported by nature's healing tools. While chronic kidney conditions may require medical supervision, **naturopathic approaches can greatly support kidney repair and overall function.**

◇ **Hot Water Therapy:**

Soaking the feet up to the knees or immersing the whole body up to the neck in warm to hot water daily for ½ to 1 hour stimulates **circulation, detoxification and healing.** This age-old therapy draws toxins away from vital organs like the kidneys and encourages better **blood flow,** allowing the body's natural repair mechanisms to function more effectively. It also relaxes the nervous system, reducing **stress-induced strain** on the kidneys.

◇ **Raw Food Diet:**

A diet rich in **fresh fruits, raw vegetables, green leafy salads, sprouts, nuts, and seeds** can help cleanse and nourish the kidneys. These natural foods are high in **antioxidants, potassium, magnesium, and enzymes** that reduce inflammation and promote healing. Hydrating fruits like watermelon, cucumber, and berries also support **kidney filtration and toxin elimination.**

◎ **"When you stop overwhelming the body with toxins and start feeding it with nature's gifts, healing becomes inevitable."**

◇ **Actionable Tip for Readers:**

- Drink a **daily detox tea** (ginger, lemon, and mint) to support digestion and detox.

4. How to Create a Healing, Plant-Rich Diet for Vitality

Adopting a plant-rich diet doesn't have to be restrictive or complicated. Instead, it's about **nourishing your body with nature's finest offerings** in an enjoyable and sustainable way.

🌱 **Steps to Transition to a Healing Diet:**

☑ **Prioritize Whole, Unprocessed Foods** – Fresh fruits, vegetables, soaked nuts, and seeds should form the foundation of every meal.

☑ **Eliminate Dairy & Animal Products** – Dairy can contribute to mucus buildup, inflammation, and digestive distress. Plant-based alternatives such as coconut milk, almond milk, and cashew cheese can provide nourishment without side effects.

☑ **Ditch Refined Sugar & Packaged Foods** – Replace with natural sweeteners like dates, raw honey, or

☑ **Include More Sprouts & Soaked Foods** – Sprouted moong, chickpeas, and soaked almonds amplify nutrient absorption and digestion.

☑ **Eat Mindfully** – Chew food slowly, eat in a peaceful environment, and express gratitude and avoid distractions while eating.

☑ **Hydrate with Natural Beverages** – Infused water, herbal teas, and coconut water instead of soda.

🔖 **Example: A nourishing plant-based plate** can include a large bowl of fresh greens, sprouts, avocado, nuts, and a lemon-tahini dressing—packed with fiber, antioxidants, and proteins.

◇ **Key Points:**

- A **plant-rich diet** is packed with nutrients that **reduce disease risk and support longevity.**

- Balance between **proteins, healthy fats, and fiber-rich carbohydrates** for sustained energy.

- The **80/20 rule:** 80% whole, plant-based foods; 20% flexibility for other foods.

◇ **Interesting Facts:**

- Studies show that plant-based diets can **reverse heart disease** and **improve insulin sensitivity.**

- The **gut microbiome thrives** on fiber from plants, promoting better digestion and immunity.

◇ **Actionable Tip for Readers:**

- Start with **one plant-based meal per day** and build up gradually.

- Morning breakfast should be of **fruits and soaked dry fruits and seeds.**

🏵 Final Thoughts

Food is our first and most powerful medicine. By making conscious choices, we can **reduce dependency on medication,** reverse chronic ailments, and experience **boundless energy and vitality.**

🌿 **A Simple Start:** Begin with small changes—swap processed snacks for nuts and fruits, drink herbal teas instead of caffeinated beverages, and incorporate more raw foods into your diet. **Your body will thank you!** 🌿

Food is not just fuel; it is the foundation of our health. Every bite we take has the potential to heal or harm. When we embrace whole, natural foods, we allow our bodies to **regenerate, detoxify, and thrive without the crutch of medications.**

Here's an easy-to-follow **meal plan** along with **simple, healing recipes** to help you incorporate a plant-based, natural healing diet into your lifestyle.

🌿 Healing Meal Plan for Natural Wellness

This meal plan is **100% plant-based,** free from dairy, animal products, refined sugar, and processed foods. It focuses on **whole, living foods** that nourish the body, reduce inflammation, and promote long-term vitality.

☺ Morning Detox & Hydration (Upon Waking)

💧 **Warm Lemon Water** – Flushes out toxins and hydrates the body.

🍵 **Herbal Detox Tea (Tulsi, Ginger, or Dandelion Tea)** – Supports liver function and digestion.

🥗 Breakfast – Energizing & Alkalizing

☑ **Option 1: Healing Fruit Bowl**

- Fresh seasonal fruits (papaya,water melon, melon, mangoes, banana, apple, pomegranate, or berries)
- Soaked almonds, walnuts, pumpkin seeds, and flaxseeds
- A drizzle of coconut water for hydration

☑ **Option 2: Soaked Nuts & Sprouts Bowl**

- Soaked and peeled almonds
- Soaked walnuts, sunflower seeds, chia seeds
- A handful of mixed sprouts (moong, chickpea, or lentil sprouts) with lemon and rock salt

☑ **Option 3: Green Detox Smoothie**

- 1 cucumber + 1 banana + 1 handful of spinach
- ½ cup coconut water
- 1 tsp chia seeds
- Blend and enjoy!

🥘 Lunch – Nourishing & Healing

☑ **Option 1: Healing Buddha Bowl**

- A mix of raw vegetables (carrot, cucumber, beetroot, cabbage,tomato, sweet potato)
- Sprouts (chickpea, moong, or lentil sprouts)
- Avocado slices for healthy fats
- Flaxseed or sesame dressing with lemon juice

☑ **Option 2: Plant-Based Millet Bowl**
- Cooked foxtail or barnyard millet
- Steamed vegetables (zucchini, bell peppers, spinach)
- Homemade coconut chutney for flavor

☑ **Option 3: Raw Vegetable Wraps**
- Cabbage or lettuce wraps filled with shredded carrots, beets, avocado, and hummus
- Sprinkled with flaxseeds and lemon dressing

☕ Mid-Afternoon (3-4 PM) – Light & Refreshing

☑ **Option 1: Coconut Water & Soaked Dates** – Rehydrates and provides natural electrolytes.

☑ **Option 2: Herbal Tea (Mint, Tulsi, or Hibiscus)** – Relieves stress and promotes digestion.

☑ **Option 3: Fresh Fruit & Nuts** – Apple with soaked walnuts or pomegranate with sunflower seeds.

🍲 Dinner – Light & Healing

☑ **Option 1: Warm Vegetable Soup with Fresh Moringa leaves**
- Carrots, pumpkin, spinach, and ginger blended into a nourishing soup
- A spoonful of **Fresh Moringa leaves** for added minerals

☑ **Option 2: Steamed Vegetables with Lemon & Herbs**
- Lightly steamed broccoli, zucchini, and mushrooms
- Sprinkled with rock salt, lemon juice, and fresh basil

☑ **Option 3: Raw Cucumber & Avocado Salad**
- Cucumber, tomatoes, avocado, coriander
- Flaxseed dressing with Himalayan salt

☽ Bedtime – Relax & Restore

☕ Turmeric & Nutmeg Herbal Drink

- 1 cup warm water
- ½ tsp turmeric powder
- A pinch of nutmeg for relaxation

✦ **Why?** This helps with deep sleep, reduces inflammation, and promotes overnight healing.

❉ Simple Healing Recipes

1. Golden Turmeric Elixir (Anti-Inflammatory Drink)

Ingredients:

☑ 1 cup warm water or coconut milk

☑ ½ tsp fresh grinded turmeric

☑ A pinch of black pepper (enhances turmeric absorption)

☑ 1 tsp raw honey (optional)

Instructions:

Mix everything well and drink before bedtime for **joint pain relief, immune boost, and deep sleep.**

2. Raw Energy Balls (Healthy Snack)

Ingredients:

☑ 1 cup soaked dates

☑ ½ cup mixed nuts (almonds, walnuts)

☑ 1 tbsp flaxseeds

☑ 1 tbsp coconut shreds

Instructions:

1. Blend all ingredients into a sticky dough.
2. Roll into small bite-sized balls.
3. Refrigerate and enjoy for an instant **energy boost!**

3. Green Detox Juice

Ingredients:

- ☑ 1 cucumber
- ☑ 1 handful spinach
- ☑ ½ lemon
- ☑ 1-inch ginger
- ☑ 1 glass coconut water

Instructions:

1. Blend everything and enjoy a refreshing, **alkalizing drink** that detoxifies and boosts energy.

🏵 Final Thoughts

These meals are **easy, healing, and deeply nourishing**. They help **reduce inflammation, improve digestion, and boost energy naturally**. Encourage yourself to start with small changes—gradually replacing processed foods with fresh, whole foods.

Conclusion of the Chapter

☑ **Summarize the key ideas:**

- Food is **powerful medicine**—healing starts on your plate.
- Focus on **anti-inflammatory and detoxifying whole foods**.
- A plant-rich diet **boosts energy, fights disease, and promotes longevity**.

◇ **Final Takeaway for Readers:**

- **Small changes lead to big results**—begin by adding more **whole, healing foods** to your diet today.

HEALING THROUGH MOVEMENT AND BREATHE

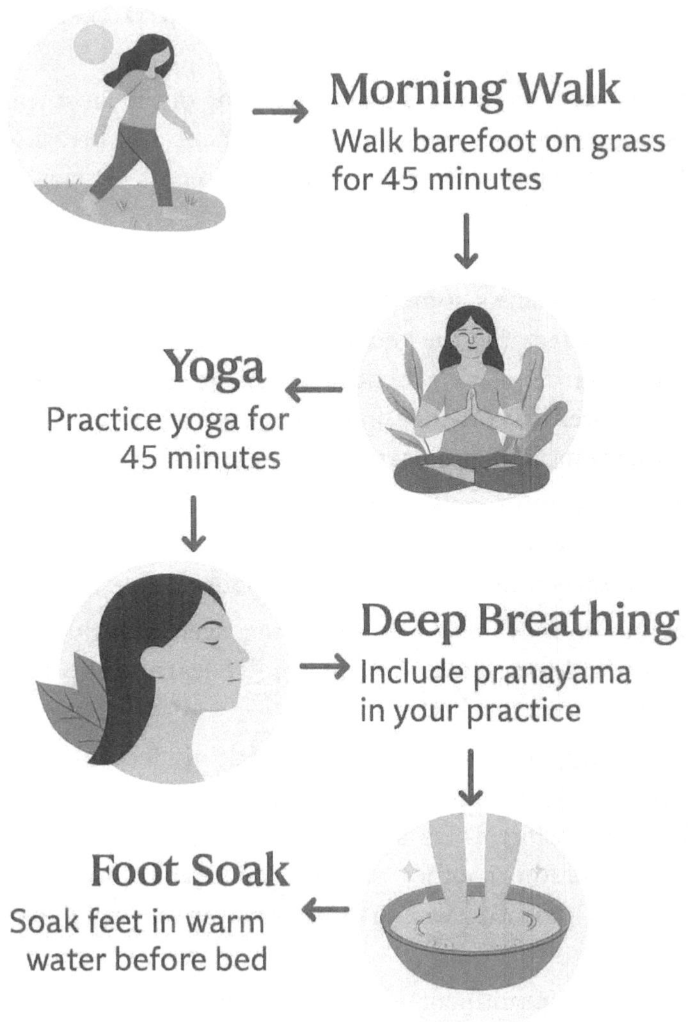

This chapter will explore how **daily movement and conscious breathing** play a vital role in healing, longevity, and overall well-being. It will guide readers on **how to use yoga, stretching, functional exercises, and breathwork** to relieve pain, reduce stress, and maintain vitality at any age.

"**Movement is medicine, and breath is the bridge between body and mind. Harness their power, and you unlock the secret to lifelong healing and vitality.**" ❉ ❧ ✤ - Reena Agarwal

❉ My Personal Practice: Moving Toward Healing Naturally

When I look back on my healing journey, one of the most transformative chapters began the moment I made movement and breathwork a daily ritual. I wasn't just searching for physical strength—I was searching for peace, vitality, and freedom from pain.

Every morning, I begin my day by walking barefoot on dewy grass for 45 minutes. There's something magical about the cool touch of the earth under my feet and the gentle warmth of the rising sun on my skin. It's not just exercise—it's grounding, a silent conversation between my body and nature. This practice, known as *earthing*, helps me feel centered, reduces inflammation, and energizes my entire being.

After this soulful walk, I move into my yoga practice. For the next 45 minutes, I stretch, exercise, and breathe. My yoga mat becomes a space of healing—where stiffness melts, pain releases, and energy flows.

I include pranayama (deep breathing exercises) that help me quiet my mind and release stress. The breath, I've learned, is a bridge to inner stillness and a powerful healer in itself.

To conclude my healing routine, I soak my feet in a basin of warm water infused with a pinch of Himalayan salt. As the warmth penetrates through my tired feet, I feel a deep sense of relaxation. This simple act supports circulation, soothes muscles, and calms my nervous system. It's become a cherished evening ritual that signals my body to rest and recharge.

This daily commitment—barefoot walking, yoga, breathwork, and warm water therapy—has not only helped me stay pain-free and flexible but has reconnected me with my own body. It's a reminder that healing doesn't always require complex treatments. Sometimes, it begins with returning to what's natural and nurturing.

My body now feels more alive, more fluid, and more at peace than it did years ago. I hope this story encourages you to create your own sacred movement routine—because healing lives in the rhythm of our breath, the stillness of our mind, and the grace of every step we take. How **consistency, simplicity, and nature can bring profound healing:**

1. The Importance of Daily Movement for Longitivity

Movement is not just about fitness—it's the language your body speaks to stay alive, young, and vibrant. Daily physical activity helps:

- **Stimulate blood circulation** and nourish every cell with oxygen and nutrients.
- **Prevent stiffness,** joint pain, and age-related immobility.
- **Boost metabolism,** which naturally declines with age.
- **Support detoxification** by moving lymph fluid and promoting sweating.
- **Improve mood and brain function** through the release of endorphins.

☞ *Studies show that just 30–45 minutes of moderate movement a day significantly reduces the risk of heart disease, diabetes, and premature aging.*

◇ **Key Points:**

- **Movement is life**—staying active prevents stiffness, pain, and disease.
- Sitting too much slows circulation, weakens muscles, and increases inflammation.
- Studies show that **people who move daily live longer and have lower risks of chronic disease.**
- **Low-impact movement** (walking, yoga, Tai Chi) is more beneficial than high-intensity exercise for long-term wellness.

◇ **Examples & Interesting Facts:**

- **The Blue Zones:** The longest-living people in the world don't go to the gym; they stay active through **daily walking, gardening, and natural movement.**

- **Muscle is anti-aging:** After age 30, we lose **3-5% of muscle per decade** unless we engage in **regular movement and strength-building exercises.**

- **10,000 Steps Myth:** Research now shows that even **4,000–5,000 steps daily** significantly reduce mortality rates.

◇ **Actionable Tip for Readers:**

- Aim for **at least 30 minutes of natural movement daily** (walking, stretching, or light exercises).

2. How Yoga, Stretching, and Functional Exercises Promote Healing

Unlike intense workouts that can exhaust the body, yoga and gentle movement nurture it. These practices:

- **Increase flexibility and joint range of motion,** reducing pain and preventing injuries.

- **Activate parasympathetic healing,** allowing your body to rest and repair.

- **Balance hormonal function,** supporting thyroid and adrenal health.

- **Tone and strengthen muscles,** especially the core and back, for better posture and support.

☞ *Poses like Cat-Cow, Downward Dog, and Child's Pose are simple yet incredibly effective for spinal health and relaxation.*

Functional movements like squats, toe touches, and shoulder rolls mirror real-life activities and are great for maintaining independence as we age.

◇ **Key Points:**

- **Yoga and stretching** improve **flexibility, circulation, and reduce joint pain.**

- **Functional exercises** (bodyweight movements, balance training) keep the body strong and prevent injuries.

- Movement improves **lymphatic drainage**, helping the body detox naturally.

◇ **Healing Benefits of Yoga & Stretching:**

- ✔ **Increases circulation** – More oxygen reaches tissues, promoting faster healing.

- ✔ **Reduces inflammation** – Gentle stretching relieves tension that contributes to pain.

- ✔ **Improves posture and mobility** – Prevents back pain, neck pain, and stiffness.

- ✔ **Boosts mood and mental clarity** – Releases feel-good hormones like **endorphins and serotonin.**

◇ **Examples & Interesting Facts:**

- **Harvard Studies show** yoga helps lower blood pressure and improves heart health.

- **Tai Chi and Qi Gong,** ancient movement practices, are scientifically proven to reduce **chronic pain and stress.**

- Stretching **before bed** can **improve sleep quality** by relaxing the nervous system.

◇ **Actionable Tip for Readers:**

- Practice a **5-minute stretching routine** every morning and night to prevent stiffness and improve flexibility.

3. The Power of Deep Breathing Techniques for Stress Reduction

Breath is life—and healing begins with it.

Chronic stress keeps the body in a "fight or flight" state, which blocks healing. Deep breathing flips that switch, helping your body relax and restore.

Breathing practices like:

- **Abdominal (diaphragmatic) breathing** – expands your lungs and calms your nervous system.

- **Box breathing** (inhale-hold-exhale-hold) – brings mental clarity and emotional balance.

- **Anulom Vilom and Bhramari pranayama** – cleanse energy channels and reduce blood pressure.

Just 10 minutes of focused breathing daily can lower cortisol, reduce anxiety, and enhance immunity.

○ **Key Points:**

- **Breathing is the fastest way to control the nervous system—** shallow breathing increases stress, while deep breathing promotes calmness.

- **The vagus nerve** (which controls relaxation) is activated through **slow, deep breaths.**

- Deep breathing improves **oxygen flow, lowers blood pressure, and enhances mental clarity.**

○ **Effective Breathing Techniques:**

- ✔ **Diaphragmatic (Belly) Breathing** – Expands the diaphragm fully, reducing stress and increasing oxygen intake.

- ✔ **4-7-8 Breathing** – Inhale for 4 seconds, hold for 7 seconds, exhale for 8 seconds (great for anxiety and sleep).

- ✔ **Box Breathing** – Inhale 4 seconds, hold 4 seconds, exhale 4 seconds, hold 4 seconds (used by Navy SEALs for focus and relaxation).

✔ **Alternate Nostril Breathing (Nadi Shodhana)** – Balances both sides of the brain, promoting emotional stability.

◇ **Examples & Interesting Facts:**
- **The longest-living yogis** credit deep breathing (Pranayama) as a key practice for **longevity and disease prevention.**
- Studies show **slow breathing (5-6 breaths per minute)** reduces anxiety and **lowers blood pressure naturally.**

◇ **Actionable Tip for Readers:**
- Try **2 minutes of deep breathing** before bed to **relieve stress and sleep better.**

4. Simple Practices to Relieve Pain and Stiffness Naturally

You don't need fancy tools—just consistent, loving care for your body. Try:
- **Walking barefoot on grass (earthing)** – reduces inflammation and improves sleep.(Detail in chapter 7)
- **Sun salutation (Surya Namaskar)** – a full-body energizer that stimulates circulation.
- **Legs-up-the-wall pose (Viparita Karani)** – relieves tired legs, back pain, and anxiety.
- **Warm water foot soaks with Epsom salts** – ease muscle tension and promote detox.
- **Foam rolling or self-massage with oil** – improves circulation and soothes tight muscles.

◇ **Key Points:**
- Chronic pain and stiffness are often due to **tight muscles, poor circulation, and stress buildup.**
- Gentle movements, proper breathing, and **hydration** can relieve pain naturally.
- **Foam rolling and massage therapy** help release **knots and tension** in the muscles.

- ◇ **Natural Pain-Relief Techniques:**
    - ✔ **Gentle stretching for 5-10 minutes** relieves back and joint pain.
    - ✔ **Hydration & electrolytes** keep muscles lubricated and prevent stiffness.
    - ✔ **Epsom salt baths** relax muscles and reduce inflammation.
    - ✔ **Self-massage or foam rolling** releases tension and promotes healing.

- ◇ **Examples & Interesting Facts:**
    - • **Dr. John Sarno's research** found that **many chronic pain cases are linked to stress and emotional tension,** not just physical injury.
    - • **Moving every hour** (even light stretching) can **prevent stiffness and pain** from prolonged sitting.

- ◇ **Actionable Tip for Readers:**
    - • **Try 5-minute mobility exercises** (neck rolls, hip openers, shoulder stretches) **every morning** to prevent pain and stiffness.

Conclusion of the Chapter

☑ **Summarize the key ideas:**

- • **Daily movement is crucial** for longevity and healing.
- • **Yoga, stretching, and deep breathing** help reduce pain, improve circulation, and lower stress.
- • **Breathwork can be a powerful tool** for activating relaxation and self-healing.

- ◇ **Final Takeaway for Readers:**
    - • **Start small but stay consistent**—move daily, stretch often, and breathe deeply for a pain-free, stress-free life.

Chapter 4

THE MIND-BODY CONNECTION AND STRESS RELIEF

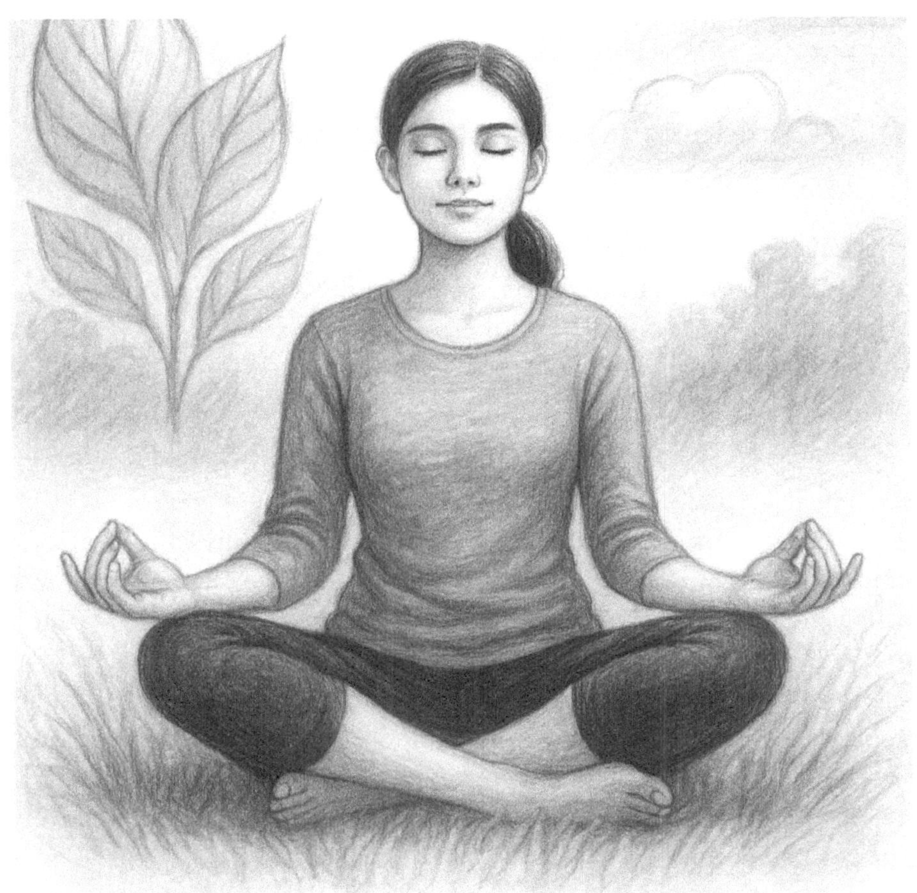

"When the mind is calm, the body follows. True healing begins not in pills, but in peace."

— Reena Agarwal

This chapter explores how **thoughts, emotions, and stress levels directly impact physical health**, and how **meditation, mindfulness, and sleep** can support healing. Readers will learn **practical, natural strategies** to reduce stress, improve resilience, and achieve mental and emotional balance.

In today's fast-paced world, **stress** has become a silent epidemic. What many don't realize is how deeply our **emotions, thoughts, and mental patterns** influence our physical health. The **mind and body** are not separate—they are intimately connected. Healing one means healing the other.

✿ My Gratitude Journey: Healing from Within

"When the mind rests, the body heals."

There was a time in my life when stress ruled my every day. Between the pressures of daily responsibilities and managing high blood pressure, I often felt like I was merely surviving, not truly living. No matter how many medicines I took, I sensed something deeper needed healing.

That's when I turned inward and discovered the missing piece—**gratitude**.

I began waking up early to sit quietly with myself, practicing simple breathing techniques and guided meditation.I began each day with a simple ritual: placing my hand over my heart and saying **"Thank you"**—for my breath, for my body, for another chance to heal. At first, it felt awkward. But slowly, I noticed something shifting inside me. My heart softened, my mind calmed, and my body began to respond. My thoughts became clearer.. I started walking barefoot in the garden, feeling the cool morning dew under my feet, letting nature calm my nervous system.

Gratitude became my daily medicine. I kept a journal, writing down 3 things I was thankful for every night. I started to see beauty in small things—a sunrise, a smile, a peaceful moment. My stress levels dropped. I slept better. I felt lighter, my mood lifted, and incredibly, even my blood pressure began to normalize.

And most importantly, I began to **heal—not just physically, but emotionally and spiritually.**

This wasn't magic. It was the natural power of aligning the mind and body through mindfulness, stillness, and a return to nature's rhythms.

Gratitude reminded me that healing isn't just about what we eat or how we move—it's about **how we feel.** And when the heart is full of appreciation, the body follows with vitality.

Today, I live free from medication—and more importantly, free from the burden of stress that once drained my joy. I want you to know that this kind of healing is available to you, too.

1. How Stress and Emotions Affect Physical Health

Chronic stress isn't just "in the mind"—it has a real, measurable impact on the body. When we're under constant pressure or emotional turmoil, our bodies respond with elevated cortisol and adrenaline. Over time, this disrupts our hormones, weakens the immune system, increases inflammation, and leads to issues like high blood pressure, digestive problems, sleep disorders, and even autoimmune conditions.

Unresolved emotions—such as grief, anger, or anxiety—can manifest physically as body aches, fatigue, or illness. For example, someone holding on to emotional pain might experience tightness in the chest, chronic back pain, or frequent headaches. When we begin to release these emotions through natural practices, we open the door to true healing.

◇ **Key Points:**
- **Stress isn't just mental—it triggers hormonal imbalances, inflammation, and disease.**
- **Chronic stress** weakens the immune system, increases blood pressure, and accelerates aging.
- Negative emotions like **anger, fear, and anxiety** release cortisol, which damages cells over time.
- The gut and brain are closely connected (**the gut produces 90% of serotonin,** affecting mood and digestion).

- ◇ **Examples & Interesting Facts:**
  - Studies show **stress contributes to 75-90% of all doctor visits,** including for headaches, heart disease, and digestive disorders.
  - People with **high stress levels are 2-3 times more likely** to develop chronic conditions like heart disease and diabetes.
  - The **Harvard "Mind Over Body" study** found that **positive emotions** (gratitude, optimism) improve heart health and boost immunity.

- ◇ **Actionable Tip for Readers:**
  - Keep a **stress journal** to identify emotional triggers and practice healthy coping strategies.

2. Meditation and Mindfulness for Healing and Resilience

Meditation is more than a practice—it is a lifestyle. Taking just 10 to 20 minutes a day to quiet the mind and breathe deeply can reduce stress levels, lower blood pressure, and activate the body's self-healing mode.

Mindfulness—being fully present in the moment—teaches us to become aware of our thoughts and feelings without judgment. It helps break the cycle of overthinking and worry. Over time, this rewires the brain, improves emotional stability, and enhances our ability to respond to life with calmness and clarity.

Practical Tip: Begin each day with a few minutes of silence. Close your eyes, focus on your breath, and repeat a calming affirmation like, *"I am safe, I am calm, I am healing."* This simple practice can shift your entire day.

- ◇ **Key Points:**
  - Meditation **reduces stress hormones, lowers blood pressure, and increases immune function.**
  - Mindfulness trains the brain to stay **present, reducing anxiety about the past or future.**

- Meditation is scientifically proven to **rewire the brain**, strengthening emotional resilience.
- **Gratitude and positive affirmations** boost mental health and enhance physical healing.

✳ How Gratitude Supports Mental and Emotional Stability:

- **Reduces stress and anxiety:** When we focus on what we're grateful for, our brain shifts from a state of fear or worry to one of peace and contentment. This calms the nervous system and reduces the production of stress hormones like cortisol.
- **Rewires the brain:** Practicing gratitude regularly can actually **change brain structure**. It increases activity in the prefrontal cortex—the area responsible for positive emotions, decision-making, and emotional regulation.
- **Improves resilience:** Grateful people tend to bounce back from challenges more easily. They're more emotionally grounded and have a broader perspective, which makes life's ups and downs easier to navigate.

⟳ How Gratitude Affects Physical Healing:

- **Strengthens the immune system:** Research has shown that people who practice gratitude regularly have **stronger immunity,** which means they're better equipped to fight off illness and recover faster from disease.
- **Lowers inflammation:** Chronic stress is linked to inflammation, the root of many modern diseases. Gratitude reduces stress, which in turn **lowers inflammation** and supports healing.
- **Improves sleep:** Grateful thoughts before bed lead to **better quality sleep,** which is essential for cellular repair, hormonal balance, and energy restoration.
- **Enhances heart health:** Gratitude is linked to **lower blood pressure, reduced heart rate,** and better circulation—an incredible benefit for those healing from chronic conditions.

☙ Simple Gratitude Practices for Healing

- ✦ Start a **daily gratitude journal** – list 3 things you're thankful for every morning or evening.

- ☺ Combine gratitude with nature – while walking barefoot on grass or during sunrise, whisper your thanks to the universe.

- 🧘 Practice **gratitude meditation** – focus on the breath and silently repeat: "Thank you for this moment, thank you for my body, thank you for healing."

- ✉ Share it – write a thank-you note or tell someone you appreciate them.

- ◎ **"Gratitude turns what we have into enough, and what we feel into healing."**

◇ Meditation Techniques for Healing:

- ✔ **Guided Meditation** – Listen to a soothing voice that directs focus on healing and relaxation.

- ✔ **Body Scan Meditation** – A mental scan of the body to release tension and pain.

- ✔ **Loving-Kindness Meditation** – Focuses on compassion and self-love, reducing emotional stress.

- ✔ **Mindful Breathing** – Simply observing the breath can calm the nervous system.

◇ Examples & Interesting Facts:

- **A UCLA study** found that people who meditate regularly have **younger-looking brains** than non-meditators.

- **Just 10 minutes of meditation daily** can reduce anxiety, improve **focus, and boost emotional balance.**

- **Monks' brains** have been studied for their extraordinary calmness and happiness, attributed to years of meditation.

◇ Actionable Tip for Readers:

- Start with **2 minutes of mindful breathing daily** and increase gradually.

3. The Role of Sleep in Disease Prevention and Cellular Repair

Sleep is one of the most underrated healing tools. During deep sleep, the body undergoes cellular repair, hormone regulation, and immune system strengthening. Poor sleep disrupts this process, making the body more vulnerable to illness and chronic stress.

Stress and mental unrest are major causes of sleep disturbances. Creating a peaceful bedtime routine—free from screens, stimulants, and negative thoughts—can significantly improve the quality of your sleep.

Natural Tips for Better Sleep:
- Drink a calming herbal tea like chamomile or tulsi.
- Practice gentle stretching or breathing before bed.
- Avoid late-night eating or digital devices.
- Listen to soft music or a sleep meditation.

◇ **Key Points:**
- Sleep is the **body's repair time**—it detoxifies the brain, regenerates cells, and balances hormones.
- **Poor sleep** weakens immunity, increases inflammation, and speeds up aging.
- **Deep sleep (REM and slow-wave sleep)** is crucial for **memory, emotional processing, and healing.**
- Sleep deprivation is linked to **weight gain, diabetes, heart disease, and depression.**

◇ **How to Improve Sleep Naturally:**
- ✔ **Follow a Sleep Schedule** – Go to bed and wake up at the same time daily.
- ✔ **Reduce Blue Light Exposure** – Avoid screens 1-2 hours before bed to support melatonin production.
- ✔ **Create a Night-time Routine** – Meditation, herbal tea, or light stretching to relax.
- ✔ **Optimize Sleep Environment** – Keep the room dark, cool, and quiet.

💤 Why Sleeping by 10 PM Supports Deep Healing

Modern science is now confirming what ancient wellness systems like Ayurveda have always known—**sleeping early is one of the most powerful tools for restoring health.**

Our bodies follow a natural rhythm known as the **circadian rhythm,** which is influenced by light and darkness. The most restorative and healing phases of sleep occur between **10 PM and 2 AM,** when the body goes into deep repair mode.

Here's what happens when you sleep by 10 PM:

- **Hormonal Balance:** The body releases melatonin, the "sleep hormone," starting around 9 PM. Sleeping by 10 PM aligns with this natural cycle, improving sleep quality and hormonal harmony.

- **Liver Detoxification:** Between 11 PM and 1 AM, the **liver** becomes most active in detoxifying the blood and processing toxins. Sleeping during this time allows it to work without interference, promoting deep cellular cleansing.

- **Cellular Repair:** Growth hormone, which is essential for **tissue repair and immune strength,** peaks during the early night hours. This helps in fighting disease and slowing down aging.

- **Mental Reset:** The brain undergoes a cleansing process, clearing out toxins linked to Alzheimer's and improving mental clarity.

🍵 Actionable Tip:

Create a calming bedtime routine starting at 9 PM—dim the lights, avoid screens, drink warm herbal tea, or read a healing book. Make your bedroom a sanctuary for rest.

> **"When you honor your body's natural rhythm, it honors you back with health, energy, and peace."**

◇ Examples & Interesting Facts:

- **Sleep deprivation affects the brain like alcohol**—reducing focus, memory, and emotional control.

- The **glymphatic system (brain's detox system)** works best during **deep sleep**, removing toxins linked to Alzheimer's.
- **Sleeping 7-9 hours** per night lowers the risk of heart disease and boosts longevity.

◇ **Actionable Tip for Readers:**

Create a **relaxing bedtime ritual** with herbal tea and deep breathing exercises.

The Circadium Rhythm

The **circadian rhythm** is your body's **natural internal clock** — a 24-hour cycle that regulates your sleep, wakefulness, hormone release, digestion, body temperature, and even mood.

Think of it like **your body's built-in schedule** that's **synchronized with nature**, especially **light and darkness**.

◇ **When it's working properly:**
- You feel energetic in the day, sleepy at night.
- Your digestion works best at certain times.
- Healing and cellular repair happen when you sleep deeply at night.
- Your body naturally detoxifies itself at night.

◇ **Key points about circadian rhythm:**
- It is **controlled by the brain's "master clock"** in the hypothalamus (specifically, the suprachiasmatic nucleus, or SCN).
- **Sunlight exposure** (especially morning light) keeps it strong and healthy.
- **Disruptions** — like sleeping late, irregular eating times, too much artificial light at night — can cause health issues like hormonal imbalance, obesity, stress, depression, and even chronic diseases.

◇ **Why it's important for healing:**

- Deep sleep at night (especially between **10 PM to 2 AM**) is when your body does **major detoxification** and **cellular repair**.

- A strong circadian rhythm **boosts immunity, balances hormones, and supports mental clarity.**

- **In simple words:**

☞ *The circadian rhythm is the rhythm of life within you. It rises with the sun, rests with the moon, and when you honor it, your body thrives naturally.*

4. Daily Habits to Stay Mentally and Emotionally Balanced

☺ **Daily Habits to Stay Mentally and Emotionally Balanced**

Healing your mind starts with consistent, nurturing habits. Small shifts in your daily routine can dramatically improve your emotional health and outlook.

Here are some powerful habits to cultivate:

- **Gratitude journaling:** Start and end the day by writing 3 things you're grateful for.

- **Digital detox:** Spend an hour each day away from screens and immerse in nature.

- **Nature breaks:** Walk barefoot, breathe in fresh air, or sit under a tree.

- **Connect meaningfully:** Talk to someone you trust or spend quality time with loved ones.

- **Laugh more:** Laughter truly is medicine. Watch something light-hearted or engage in activities that bring joy.

◇ **Key Points:**

- Emotional balance comes from **healthy daily habits**—not just one-time stress relief activities.

- Small practices like **gratitude, journaling, and spending time in nature** have lasting mental benefits.
- Building a **resilient mindset** helps handle challenges without chronic stress responses.

◇ **Simple Daily Practices for Emotional Well-being:**
  - ✔ **Gratitude Journaling** – Writing down three things you're grateful for shifts focus to positivity.
  - ✔ **Spending Time in Nature** – Walking outside reduces cortisol and boosts serotonin.
  - ✔ **Limiting Social Media** – Less screen time reduces anxiety and mental fatigue.
  - ✔ **Connecting with Loved Ones** – Social connections enhance emotional resilience and happiness.

◇ **Examples & Interesting Facts:**
  - **Forest bathing (Shinrin-Yoku)** in Japan has been scientifically proven to **reduce stress and improve immune function.**
  - **Writing down worries before bed** helps clear the mind and improve sleep quality.
  - **Hugging or physical touch** increases **oxytocin,** the "love hormone," which reduces stress.

◇ **Actionable Tip for Readers:**
  - Start a **5-minute gratitude practice** each morning to shift into a positive mindset.

Conclusion of the Chapter

☑ Summarize the key ideas:
  - **Your mind and emotions shape your physical health.**
  - **Meditation and mindfulness** are powerful tools for healing and stress relief.
  - **Sleep is essential** for longevity and disease prevention.

- Daily habits like gratitude, nature exposure, and social connections promote lasting emotional balance.

◇ **Final Takeaway for Readers:**

- Small shifts in **thoughts, breathing, and daily routines** can create **profound healing effects** on both mind and body.

🏵 Final Thought

When the mind is calm, the body follows. And when both are in harmony, healing becomes effortless. In this chapter, we've explored how your thoughts, emotions, sleep, and daily habits form the emotional backbone of your health. Embrace the stillness within, and watch your body flourish.

✿ Daily Affirmation:

"I breathe in calm. I breathe out stress. My body is safe, strong, and healing."

Chapter 5

NATURE'S PHARMACY – HERBS AND NATURAL REMEDIES

"In every leaf, root, and flower lies nature's quiet remedy—gentle, powerful, and waiting to heal."

– Reena Agarwal

Nature has always offered powerful healing tools—long before modern medicine. From herbs and oils to home remedies passed down through generations, this chapter invites you to explore the age-old wisdom of healing with nature's gifts.

This chapter explores the **power of nature's medicine cabinet**, showing readers how to use **herbs, essential oils, and natural remedies** to boost immunity, relieve pain, and prevent illness. It also guides them on creating their **own natural medicine cabinet** for everyday health concerns.

1. Healing Herbs for Immunity, Digestion, and Inflammation

🌱 **Key Herbs:**

- **Tulsi (Holy Basil):** Known as the **"Queen of Herbs,"** it boosts immunity, reduces stress, and supports respiratory health.

- **Ginger:** A natural anti-inflammatory, great for digestion, nausea, and joint pain.

- **Turmeric (Curcumin):** A powerful antioxidant that fights inflammation and supports brain and heart health.

- **Ashwagandha:** An adaptogen that calms the nervous system and strengthens immunity.

- **Peppermint:** Soothes digestive troubles, reduces bloating, and cools inflammation.

◇ **Key Points:**

- Herbs have been used for **centuries in Ayurveda, Traditional Chinese Medicine (TCM), and Indigenous healing practices.**

- Many pharmaceutical drugs originate from plant compounds, proving the potency of **natural medicine.**

- Some herbs are **anti-inflammatory, antibacterial, antiviral, or adaptogenic,** helping the body resist stress.

◇ **Powerful Healing Herbs:**

- ✔ **For Immunity:** Echinacea (fights colds), Elderberry (antiviral), Astragalus (immune booster).

- ✔ **For Digestion:** Ginger (soothes nausea), Peppermint (relieves bloating), Fennel (aids digestion).

- ✔ **For Inflammation:** Turmeric (curcumin reduces pain), Boswellia (anti-arthritis), Green Tea (rich in antioxidants).

- ✔ **For Stress & Sleep:** Ashwagandha (lowers cortisol), Chamomile (calming), Lemon Balm (relieves anxiety).

◇ **Examples & Interesting Facts:**

- **Echinacea boosts white blood cells,** helping fight infections faster.

- **Curcumin in fresh turmeric is as effective as some pain relievers** in reducing joint pain.

- **Garlic has natural antibiotic properties,** often called "nature's penicillin."

- **Ginger** is one of nature's most powerful healing roots.

- Many of these herbs have been used for over 3,000 years in **Ayurveda and traditional Chinese medicine.**

✤ Healing Properties of Fresh Turmeric Root (Curcumin)

Fresh curcumin, the active compound found in turmeric root, is a golden gem of natural healing. When used in its fresh form, it retains even more potent therapeutic properties compared to its dried or powdered counterparts. Here's an overview of its healing benefits and practical uses:

◇ Powerful Anti-inflammatory:

- Curcumin blocks inflammatory molecules, making it highly effective in reducing chronic inflammation—a root cause of many diseases including arthritis, heart disease, and metabolic issues.

◇ Natural Antioxidant:

- It neutralizes free radicals and stimulates the body's own antioxidant enzymes, helping to slow aging and prevent oxidative stress-related damage.

◇ Supports Liver Detox:

- Curcumin enhances liver function by promoting bile flow, which helps the body to detox naturally and more efficiently.

◇ Boosts Immunity:

- It activates immune cells, increases resistance against infection, and supports the body's natural defense systems.

◇ Aids Digestion:

- Curcumin stimulates digestive enzymes, reducing bloating, gas, and indigestion while supporting a healthy gut microbiome.

◇ Promotes Brain Health:

- Curcumin boosts levels of brain-derived neurotrophic factor (BDNF), supporting memory, mood, and overall cognitive health.

◇ Natural Pain Reliever:

- Its analgesic properties can ease joint pain, menstrual cramps, and general body aches.

♟ How to Use Fresh Curcumin in Daily Life

♟ 1. Golden Morning Shot:

- Blend a small piece (1 inch) of fresh turmeric root with lemon juice, a pinch of black pepper (enhances absorption), and honey or coconut water.

- Drink on an empty stomach to kickstart detox and boost immunity.

♟ 2. Turmeric Paste:

- Grate fresh turmeric and mix with a little water or oil to make a paste.

- Use topically for minor wounds, inflammation, or skin infections (antibacterial and wound-healing).

♟ 3. Add to Smoothies or Juices:

- Blend a knob of turmeric root into vegetable juices or fruit smoothies for an earthy, spicy kick and enhanced health benefits.

♟ 4. Herbal Tea or Decoction:

- Simmer slices of turmeric root in water with ginger, cinnamon, and a dash of black pepper. Strain and sip for soothing relief from colds or inflammation.

♟ 5. Healing Turmeric Milk:

- Grate turmeric into warm plant-based milk with a pinch of black pepper and cinnamon—especially helpful before bed for joint pain and sleep.

♟ 6. Cooking & Curries:

- Grated turmeric can be added to soups, stews, lentils, and curries for both color and medicinal value.

❄ Your Ideal Naturopathic Curcumin Booster

Here's a healing drink idea:

Blend 1 inch fresh turmeric, a small pinch of black pepper, soaked almonds or coconut water, and lemon juice. Strain and drink first thing in the morning to enhance curcumin's bioavailability and absorption in the body. ☺

❀ Healing Properties of Ginger

Ginger contains gingerols, which are natural anti-inflammatory compounds. These help reduce swelling and pain, especially in conditions like:

- Arthritis
- Joint pain
- Muscle soreness

Ginger stimulates digestion and relieves various gastrointestinal discomforts:

- Nausea and vomiting (especially morning sickness or motion sickness)
- Indigestion
- Gas and bloating

Ginger has natural antibacterial, antiviral, and antioxidant properties that:

- Strengthen the immune system
- Help fight infections
- Prevent cold and flu

☑ Tip: Add grated ginger to your herbal teas or warm water with lemon and honey during seasonal changes.

Ginger acts as a natural analgesic. It's effective in relieving pain:

- Headaches
- Menstrual cramps
- Muscle soreness

Ginger may help improve insulin sensitivity and lower blood sugar levels, supporting:

- Diabetes prevention
- Balanced energy levels

Ginger supports heart health by:

- Improving circulation
- Reducing cholesterol levels
- Lowering blood pressure

☑ Tip: Use **ginger in daily cooking or juice it with carrots and beets** for heart health.

♥ Quote:

"**Ginger is a gift from the Earth – warming, cleansing, and full of life-giving energy.**"

◇ **Actionable Tip for Readers:**

- Start the day with **warm herbal tea**—like **ginger + tulsi + turmeric**—to awaken your digestion, energize your immunity, reduce inflammation and support digestion.

2. Essential Oils for Relaxation, Pain Relief, and Energy

✿ **Key Essential Oils:**

- **Lavender:** Calms anxiety, supports sleep, and reduces tension headaches.
- **Eucalyptus:** Clears the respiratory tract and relieves sinus congestion.
- **Peppermint Oil:** Provides energy, focus, and instant relief from headaches or nausea.
- **Frankincense:** Supports cellular health, immunity, and spiritual clarity.
- **Lemon or Orange Oil:** Boosts mood and detoxes the body when inhaled or applied topically (diluted).

◇ **Key Points:**

- Essential oils are **highly concentrated plant extracts** that can affect mood, pain levels, and energy.

- Aromatherapy can **stimulate the brain's limbic system**, influencing emotions and memory.

- Oils can be **inhaled, applied topically, or added to baths and diffusers.**

◇ **Best Essential Oils for Healing:**

- ✔ **For Relaxation & Stress Relief:** Lavender (calms the mind), Frankincense (reduces anxiety), Bergamot (uplifts mood).

- ✔ **For Pain Relief:** Peppermint (eases headaches), Eucalyptus (soothes muscle pain), Clove (great for toothaches).

- ✔ **For Energy & Focus:** Rosemary (enhances memory), Citrus oils (boosts alertness), Peppermint (refreshes).

- ✔ **For Sleep:** Chamomile (calming), Vetiver (deep relaxation), Cedarwood (improves sleep quality).

◇ **Examples & Interesting Facts:**

- Lavender oil has been clinically proven to **reduce anxiety as effectively as medication.**

- **Peppermint oil on the temples** can **relieve headaches within minutes.**

- **Citrus scents like lemon and orange** can **boost energy and improve mood** instantly.

- Inhalation of essential oils stimulates the **limbic system, the brain's emotional center,** directly influencing **mood and health.**

◇ **Actionable Tip for Readers:**

- Diffuse **lavender and frankincense** oil in your bedroom before sleep or dab peppermint oil on temples to ease fatigue to promote restful sleep

3. Home Remedies for Common Ailments

⚕ Natural Solutions:

- **For Headaches:** Apply peppermint oil to the temples and rest in a dark room.
- **For Colds & Cough:** Mix turmeric, honey, and black pepper in warm water
- **For Joint Pain:** Massage with warm sesame oil infused with ginger or eucalyptus.
- **For Indigestion:** Drink fennel seed tea after meals.
- **For Sore Throat:** Gargle with warm salt water and turmeric.

◇ Key Points:

- Natural remedies can address **everyday health concerns** without synthetic drugs.
- Herbs, essential oils, and food-based solutions can be combined for **powerful relief.**
- Simple household ingredients like **honey, apple cider vinegar, and salt** have healing properties.

◇ Natural Remedies for Common Ailments:

- ✔ **Headaches** – Peppermint oil on temples, magnesium-rich foods, hydration with lemon water.
- ✔ **Colds & Flu** – Elderberry syrup, honey and ginger tea, steam inhalation with eucalyptus oil.
- ✔ **Joint Pain** – Turmeric with black pepper, Epsom salt baths, Boswellia supplements.
- ✔ **Indigestion & Bloating** – Fennel or ginger tea, apple cider vinegar before meals, peppermint capsules.
- ✔ **Insomnia** – Warm chamomile tea, magnesium rich foods, lavender pillow spray.
- ✔ **Stress & Anxiety** – Deep breathing with frankincense, adaptogenic herbs like ashwagandha, journaling.

◇ **Examples & Interesting Facts:**

- **Honey and cinnamon** together have antimicrobial properties that support immunity.
- **A teaspoon of apple cider vinegar before meals** can improve digestion and reduce bloating.
- **Ginger is as effective as ibuprofen** for relieving menstrual cramps.
- Many of these **home remedies** work by **enhancing circulation, reducing inflammation, and balancing internal energies.**

◇ **Actionable Tip for Readers:**

- Create a "Remedy Box" with go-to items like rock salt, ginger, raw honey, turmeric, and eucalyptus oil for quick relief at home.

4. How to Create a Natural Medicine Cabinet at Home

🛒 **Must-Haves for Every Natural Home:**

- **Dry herbs:** Tulsi, ginger, peppermint, chamomile
- **Spices:** Turmeric, cinnamon, clove, black pepper
- **Essential oils:** Lavender, eucalyptus, lemon, peppermint
- **Natural items:** Rock salt, raw honey, fresh aloe vera gel, coconut oil
- **Tools:** Mortar & pestle, small glass jars, dropper bottles, diffuser

◇ **Key Points:**

- Stocking a home **apothecary with essential herbs, oils, and remedies** ensures preparedness for minor health issues.
- Keeping high-quality, **organic, and properly stored** ingredients maintains their potency.
- Having a balance of **immune boosters, pain relievers, digestive aids, and stress reducers** creates a well-rounded kit.

◇ **Must-Have Items for a Natural Medicine Cabinet:**

- ✔ **Herbs & Teas:** Turmeric, ginger, chamomile, echinacea, peppermint.
- ✔ **Essential Oils:** Lavender (sleep), Tea Tree (antibacterial), Peppermint (pain relief).
- ✔ **Natural Supplements:** Magnesium (relaxation), Probiotics (gut health), Vitamin D (immune support).
- ✔ **Healing Foods:** Honey, garlic, coconut oil.
- ✔ **Topical Remedies:** Fresh Aloe vera gel (skin healing), Paste of fresh green leaves (bruises), Witch hazel (soothing skin).

◇ **Examples & Interesting Facts:**

- **Fresh Aloe vera can heal burns faster** than conventional creams.
- **Oil pulling with coconut oil** can reduce oral bacteria and improve gum health.
- **Wheat grass juice** also helps to improve gum and oral health
- **Arnica gel and Fresh Aloe vera has been found to be as effective as ibuprofen** for muscle pain and bruises.
- Store your **herbs and oils** in a cool, dark place in airtight containers to preserve potency.

◇ **Actionable Tip for Readers:**

- Start building a **small natural medicine cabinet** with **5 essential items**: ginger, turmeric, lavender oil, honey, and magnesium.
- Make simple herbal blends, like "Immunity Tea" (ginger, tulsi, cinnamon) and keep them ready in small jars. Label them beautifully and keep your cabinet visually inspiring!

Conclusion of the Chapter

☑ Summarize the key ideas:

- **Herbs, essential oils, and home remedies** can be as powerful as modern medicine for everyday health concerns.
- **Nature offers solutions for immunity, digestion, pain relief, and stress reduction.**
- A well-stocked **natural medicine cabinet** can provide healing support at home.

◇ **Final Takeaway for Readers:**

- **Start simple but stay consistent**—integrate herbs, oils, and remedies into daily life for long-term well-being.

🌼 Closing Thought:

"Let food be thy medicine and medicine be thy food."

– Hippocrates

Nature's remedies are not just about healing symptoms—they bring us back to balance and wholeness, restoring health from the roots.

Chapter 6

DETOXIFICATION AND CLEANSING FOR VITALITY

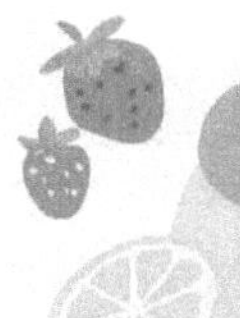

1 Why Regular Detoxing is Essctial for Lifelong Wellness

- Toxins bulid up from diet & environment
- Stress weakens detox functions
- Cleansing prevents disease & boost cnergy

Ways to Practice:
- Avaid sugar & processed foods
- Eat raw fruits & sprouts

Actionable Tip:
Start a "detox journal."

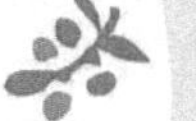

2 The best Ways to Cleanse Your Body Naturally—Foods. Herbs, and Practices

- Detox foods:
  Fruits: paoya watermelon
- Greens: chia chla. pumpkin
- Herbs: triphala mint

Detox Practices
Dry brushing
Sunnbathing

Actionable Fact:
Moming detox rotne

Interessting Fact:
- Create a **morning** detox routine: warm lemon watar + yoga

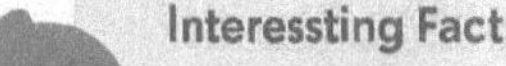

3 Safe and Simple Detox Routine for Daily Life

- Daily detox rituals Fruit only breakfasts
- Green juice
- Evening foot soaks

Anteresting Fact:
Choose one **detox** ritual for 7 days

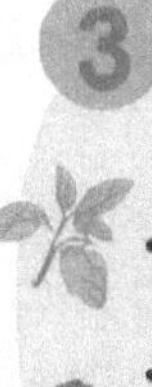

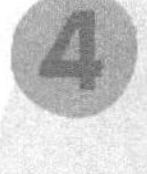

4 The Role of Fasting and Hydration in Deep Healing

- Fasting allows body to repair — water
- Water flushes toxins from system

Ways to Practice:
- Fruit or juice fasting
- Drink 2.5-3 L.a. day aer aday

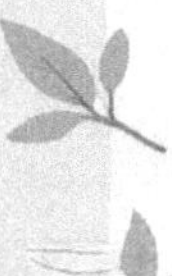

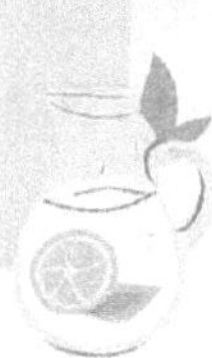

"Your body is your sacred home—cleanse it with the gifts of nature, and it will reward you with boundless energy, clarity, and vibrant health."

"One green juice a day keeps the doctor away. For me, that's something that I really try to have everyday or make every day" - Karolina Kurkova

❅ My Detox Journey: Reclaiming Energy and Inner Peace

"How Detoxing Gave Me Back My Energy, Clarity, and Calm"

A few years ago, despite eating healthier than before, I still felt sluggish, foggy, and emotionally overwhelmed. I realized I needed a deeper level of cleansing—one that would help me reset both physically and mentally. That's when I discovered the power of **fruit fasting and deep hydration.**

For three consecutive days, I switched to a fruit-only diet—mainly melons, papayas, and oranges—and increased my water intake significantly. To support the cleanse, I started each morning with warm lemon water, followed by fresh coconut water and green juice. I rested more, practiced gentle yoga, and spent quiet time in nature.

By day three, something magical happened. My energy surged, my mind felt clear, and I experienced an emotional calm I hadn't felt in years. My skin glowed, my digestion improved, and I felt lighter—not just in body but in spirit. That detox reset helped me understand how deeply our bodies crave simplicity, purity, and natural rhythms.

Today, I incorporate regular mini-detoxes and juice days into my lifestyle—not for weight loss, but to maintain balance and allow my body to heal and thrive. It's one of the most empowering self-care rituals I follow.

"When we stop overwhelming the body, it begins to speak—and it always speaks in the language of healing."

1. Why Regular Detoxing Is Essential for Lifelong Wellness

☑ Key Points:

- **Toxic Load:** Daily exposure to environmental pollutants, processed food, stress, and synthetic chemicals overwhelms the liver and kidneys.

- **Signs You Need a Detox:** Chronic fatigue, skin issues, digestive problems, bloating, frequent headaches, brain fog, and low immunity.

- **Benefits of Regular Detoxing:** Increased energy, mental clarity, glowing skin, better digestion, hormone balance, reduced inflammation, and overall vitality.

- When **detox organs (liver, kidneys, skin, lungs)** are overwhelmed, symptoms appear: fatigue, brain fog, skin issues, bloating, or illness.

ⴲ Ways to Practice:

- Reduce or eliminate refined sugar, dairy, and processed foods.

- Introduce raw foods like fruits and sprouts.

- Create seasonal detox days with mono fruit meals or light soups.

⚲ Interesting Fact:

- The liver regenerates itself! A clean diet can help rebuild liver cells in just 30–45 days.(details given in chapter 2)

- The body has five main detox pathways: liver, lungs, kidneys, skin, and colon. If one is sluggish, the others get overloaded.

⬭ Actionable Tip:

- **Start a "detox journal."** Note how you feel before and after a week of clean eating—observe changes in energy, digestion, skin, and sleep.

2. The Best Ways to Cleanse Your Body Naturally—Foods, Herbs, and Practices

☑ **Key Points:**

- Nature provides powerful cleansing tools—no chemicals or harsh products needed.
- Specific foods, herbs, and lifestyle practices help remove toxins and renew the body.

🌱 **Natural Detox Foods:**

- **Leafy greens** (spinach, coriander, moringa, wheatgrass) support liver function.
- **Fruits** (papaya, citrus, pomegranate, apples) for fiber and antioxidants.
- **Raw juices** (celery, beetroot, cucumber, lemon-ginger) to flush toxins.
- **Soaked nuts & seeds** for gentle nourishment.

Detox Herbs:

- **Triphala, milk thistle, dandelion root,** and **turmeric** cleanse the liver and colon.
- **Neem** and **giloy** strengthen immunity.

Detoxifying Practices:

- **Dry brushing** for lymphatic flow.
- **Tongue scraping** to eliminate toxins.
- **Steam therapy, sun bathing,** and **herbal baths**– Stimulates vitamin D and internal cleansing
- **Walking barefoot (Earthing)** – Grounds excess positive ions (inflammation)
- **Warm water with lemon** – A gentle daily flush

💡 **Interesting Fact:**

- The skin eliminates nearly **1 pound of waste daily** through sweat. Dry brushing + movement enhances this natural detox!

○ **Actionable Tip:**

Morning Detox Routine: Start your day with warm lemon water + 20 minutes of yoga or stretching to activate detox organs.

3. Safe and Simple Detox Routines for Daily Life

☑ **Key Points:**

- Detoxing doesn't have to be drastic—it can be part of your daily rhythm.
- Small, consistent habits make the biggest impact over time.

🌱 **Examples of Daily Detox Rituals:**

- **Fruit-only breakfast** – Cleanses the digestive tract
- **Green juice or smoothie** – Boosts nutrient absorption and alkalizes the body
- **Evening foot soak in warm water + rock salt** – Pulls toxins from the body
- **Herbal teas** – Ginger-fennel, cumin-coriander, or tulsi to flush toxins
- **Evening walk under the moonlight** – Calms the nervous system and resets biorhythm

Daily Detox Habits:

- Start your day with **warm water + lemon.**
- **Intermittent fasting** (e.g., 14-16 hours fast) to allow the body time to cleanse.(details given in chapter 2)
- **Oil pulling** with cold-pressed sesame or coconut oil.
- **One raw meal** per day (fruit bowl, salad, sprouts).
- **Avoiding** white sugar, refined flour, dairy, and packaged snacks.

💡 **Interesting Fact:**

- According to Ayurveda, **digestion is strongest between 10 a.m. to 2 p.m.**—eating your largest meal (fresh fruits, salads and soaked dry fruits) during this window supports natural detox.

💬 **Actionable Tip:**

Choose **one detox ritual to practice for 7 days**—like fruit breakfast or nightly foot soak—and observe how your body responds.

Personal Touch Idea: Share your daily detox routine—perhaps your lemon water ritual, daily green juice, or raw salad meals.

4. The Role of Fasting and Hydration in Deep Healing

☑ **Key Points:**

- Fasting gives the digestive system a break so the body can focus on healing and regeneration.
- Hydration is essential to flush out released toxins during fasting and cleansing.

🌱 **Ways to Practice:**

- **Intermittent fasting or autophagy**(12–16 hrs daily) – A gentle start.(details given in chapter 2)
- **24-hour fruit fast** once a week – Papaya, melons, or citrus fruits
- **Juice fasting** – 1–3 days with fresh veggie and fruit juices
- **Herbal infusions & water therapy** – Drink 2.5–3L/day (add mint, lemon, or cucumber)
- **Fasting:**
  - Stimulates **autophagy** (the body's cellular cleaning process).
  - Gives the digestive system a rest, redirecting energy toward repair.
  - Ancient and natural healing method practiced in every culture.
- **Types of Fasting:**
  - Intermittent fasting, juice fasting, fruit fasting, or weekly 24-hour water fast.

- Hydration:
  - **At least 8-10 glasses of pure water daily** to flush out toxins.
  - Add **natural electrolytes**—like a pinch of rock salt, lemon, or soaked basil seeds.
  - **Coconut water and cucumber juice** are deeply hydrating.

💡 Interesting Fact:

- Just 1-2% **dehydration** can reduce cognitive function and energy levels. Hydration is critical during any detox protocol.
- During fasting, the body enters a repair mode called **autophagy**—damaged cells are broken down and recycled, promoting longevity.

💬 Actionable Tip:

Start with a **"fruit-only dinner" twice a week** to ease into fasting. Follow it with a calming tea like chamomile or ginger.

🕸 Bonus Add-Ons:

- **A Gentle 3-Day Detox Plan:**
  - Day 1: Fruit & juice cleanse
  - Day 2: Light khichdi + steamed veggies
  - Day 3: Raw salad + coconut water

🧠 Key Points:

- **The body is self-cleaning—if we allow it:** Our liver, kidneys, lungs, skin, and lymphatic system naturally detoxify the body, but modern lifestyles overload them.
- **Toxic overload is real:** Pesticides, processed foods, pollution, stress, and poor sleep all contribute to toxin buildup.
- **Detoxing is not a trend—it's a necessity:** Regular cleansing helps prevent disease, improves energy, clears the skin, and enhances mental clarity.
- **Gentle, daily detoxing is better than harsh fads.**

🌿 Best Ways to Cleanse Your Body Naturally

1. **Detoxifying Foods:**

   Fruits: Papaya, oranges, watermelon, pomegranate, apples

   Veggies: Leafy greens, beets, cucumbers, carrots

   Herbs: Cilantro (heavy metal detox), mint, parsley

   Seeds & Nuts: Soaked almonds, chia, flax

   Healing drinks: Coconut water, lemon water, green juices, fresh vegetable broth

2. **Powerful Detox Herbs:**

   Triphala: supports digestion and bowel regularity

   Milk Thistle: rejuvenates the liver

   Turmeric: anti-inflammatory and liver-protective

   Neem: blood purifier

   Dandelion root: supports liver and kidneys

3. **Detox Practices:**

   - **Dry brushing:** stimulates lymphatic drainage
   - **Sweating (via sun, yoga, or warm baths):** helps eliminate toxins
   - **Breathwork:** oxygenates the body and releases carbon dioxide (a waste product)
   - **Hot foot soaks:** relax muscles and support detox through the feet
   - **Sun exposure & grounding:** restore natural balance and improve circulation

🔄 Safe & Simple Detox Routines for Daily Life:

- **Morning detox ritual:** Start the day with warm lemon water + gentle yoga
- **Fruit-only breakfast:** High-fiber fruits help clean the digestive tract
- **Juice therapy:** A glass of green juice mid-morning or evening

- **Weekly mono-fruit fast:** One day a week with only melons or papaya
- **Evening herbal tea cleanse:** Triphala or ginger-fennel tea

✦ Interesting Facts:

- **The skin is the largest detox organ** – That's why breakouts can signal inner toxicity.
- **Your body detoxes most efficiently between 10 p.m. and 2 a.m.** – So restful sleep is crucial for natural cleansing.(Details in chapter 4)
- **70–80% of the immune system lives in the gut** – Detoxing the digestive tract supports immunity.
- **Grounding (walking barefoot) helps reduce inflammation** by discharging built-up positive ions (electrical charge) into the Earth.(Details in chapter 3)

☑ Actionable Tips for Readers:

- ☺ **Start small:** Replace one meal with a fruit bowl or smoothie.
- 🧘 **Choose one detox ritual per day:** Try a foot soak or dry brushing.
- ☕ **Drink healing teas at night:** Ginger-turmeric or fennel-coriander-cumin mix.
- 🗓 **Create a 3-day seasonal cleanse:** Stick to hydrating foods, herbal teas, sunbathing, and rest.
- 📖 **Keep a detox journal:** Track how you feel before and after cleansing days.

THE HEALING POWER OF SUNLIGHT, WATER, AND EARTH

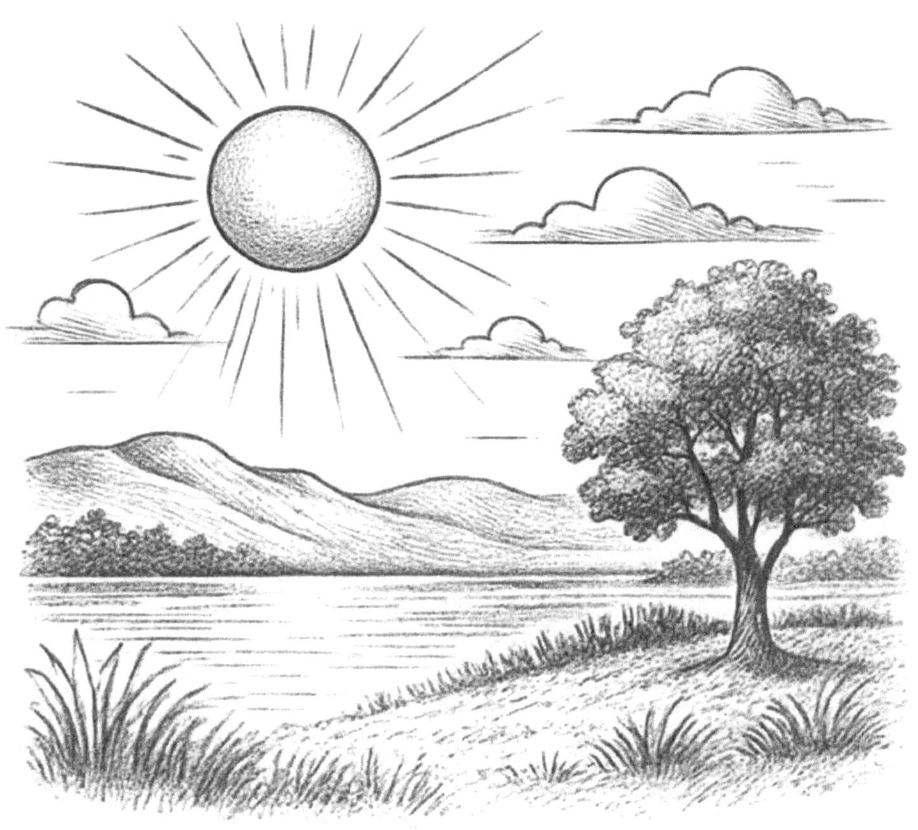

☺ Inspirational Quote:

"The sun, the soil, and the streams—nature's silent healers— offer us vitality, peace, and renewal. We only need to remember to return to them."

– Reena Agarwal

This chapter explores how **natural elements—sunlight, water, and the Earth itself—support healing, reduce stress, and enhance longevity.** Readers will learn how to harness these powerful forces for optimal health.

❄ Personal Story: My Healing Journey with Sun, Water & Earth

There was a time in my life when I felt disconnected—from my body, from peace, and from the natural world. Stress, illness, and the noise of modern life clouded my vitality. But everything changed when I made a conscious decision to return to nature.

Each morning, I began walking barefoot on the cool grass, letting the warmth of the morning sun kiss my skin. This simple practice— grounding and sunbathing—became my daily ritual of healing. I would breathe deeply, feeling the pulse of the Earth beneath my feet and the calm of the sky above.

Hydration, too, played its role. I started every day with warm lemon water, sipped fresh coconut water, and filled my plate with hydrating fruits. My body responded. The heaviness lifted. My energy returned.

Nature, with its gentle yet powerful touch, began to restore me— physically, emotionally, and spiritually. I realized that healing doesn't have to be complicated. Sometimes, all we need is to step outside, take a breath, and allow the Earth to do what it does best—bring us back into balance.

1. ⬡ The Benefits of Sun Exposure for Vitamin D and Overall Health

Sunlight is nature's most powerful and free healing source.

Sunlight is one of the **most natural, powerful, and free sources of healing** available to us — yet it's often overlooked in modern life. Let's explore how sunlight nurtures and transforms our health at multiple levels:

⬡ Benefits of Sunlight for Health

1. **Boosts Vitamin D Production:**
   - When sunlight hits your skin, it triggers the production of **vitamin D,** often called the "sunshine vitamin."
   - Vitamin D is crucial for **strong bones, immunity, mental health,** and **prevention of chronic diseases** like diabetes, heart disease, and certain cancers.

2. **Strengthens Immunity:**
   - Adequate sunlight exposure enhances the **immune system,** helping the body fight infections and inflammation naturally.

3. **Regulates Mood and Fights Depression:**
   - Sunlight stimulates the release of **serotonin,** the "feel-good" hormone that improves mood, focus, and calmness.
   - Lack of sunlight can lead to **Seasonal Affective Disorder (SAD),** a type of depression linked to reduced light exposure.

4. **Supports Healthy Sleep Patterns:**
   - Morning sunlight helps **synchronize your circadian rhythm,** signaling your body when to wake up and when to produce melatonin for restful sleep at night.

5. **Improves Heart Health:**
   - Sunlight can cause **natural dilation of blood vessels,** lowering blood pressure and improving heart function.

6. **Promotes Detoxification:**
   - Sunlight helps activate the **lymphatic system,** enhancing the removal of toxins and supporting deeper body cleansing.

7. **Enhances Skin Health (in Moderation):**
   - Controlled exposure to sunlight can help in healing **eczema, psoriasis, acne,** and other skin disorders.
   - It increases production of antimicrobial peptides, boosting the skin's natural defense barrier.

8. **Supports Metabolic Health:**
   - Some research suggests sunlight exposure may help regulate **insulin sensitivity** and **prevent metabolic syndrome.**

☺ **How Much Sunlight Do You Need?**
   - **15–30 minutes a day,** preferably in the morning, on bare skin (like arms, face, and legs), without sunscreen for a short period.
   - The exact time needed varies based on **skin tone, geographic location,** and **season.**
   - Morning sunlight (before 10 a.m.) is the safest and most beneficial.

🐾 **Personal Note:**

In my healing journey, **early morning sunlight walks** became medicine for my mind and body. Just 20 minutes of morning light each day not only **lifted my spirits** but also **accelerated my physical healing,** bringing me clarity, energy, and a deep sense of connection to life.

✦ **Final Thought:**

   "The sun doesn't just light up the world — it lights up your health from the inside out."

By embracing the healing rays of sunlight consciously and respectfully, you awaken the body's natural brilliance to heal, energize, and thrive.

◇ **Key Points:**
- Sunlight is the **primary source of Vitamin D,** essential for **strong bones, immunity, mood regulation, and hormone balance.**
- Moderate sun exposure **reduces the risk of depression, heart disease, and autoimmune disorders.**
- Sunlight **syncs the body's circadian rhythm,** improving sleep and energy levels.
- **Overuse of sunscreen and indoor lifestyles have led to a global Vitamin D deficiency crisis.**

◇ **How to Get Safe Sun Exposure:**
- ✔ **Expose skin for 10-30 minutes daily** (depending on skin tone and location).
- ✔ **Morning sunlight (before 10 AM) is ideal** for resetting the body clock and reducing stress.
- ✔ **Avoid excessive midday sun,** but don't block all UV exposure.
- ✔ **Foods that enhance Vitamin D absorption:** mushrooms, avocado,etc.

◇ **Examples & Interesting Facts:**
- **80% of people worldwide are Vitamin D deficient,** leading to increased risks of chronic illness.
- **Sunlight boosts serotonin,** making it nature's natural antidepressant.
- **A Harvard study found that adequate sunlight exposure reduces the risk of certain cancers.**

◇ **Interesting Fact:**
- Just **15–30 minutes of sunlight exposure** on the skin (without sunscreen) a few times a week can meet your body's vitamin D needs, depending on skin type and location.

◇ **Example:**
  - In Japan, "shinrin-yoku" or "forest bathing" incorporates sunlight and nature exposure to reduce cortisol levels and enhance emotional well-being.

◇ **Actionable Tip for Readers:**
  - Spend **20 minutes outdoors daily** without sunglasses to absorb full-spectrum light.
  - Aim for **early morning sunlight**—it's gentler, boosts your mood, and helps regulate your circadian rhythm for better sleep.

🥑 **Plant-Based Foods that Support Vitamin D Absorption:**

1. **Avocados:**
   - Rich in healthy fats which help in **absorbing fat-soluble vitamins** like vitamin D.

2. **Nuts and Seeds:** (especially **walnuts, almonds, chia seeds, flaxseeds**)
   - Provide **good fats** and **magnesium,** both essential for vitamin D metabolism.

3. **Coconut:** (fresh coconut, coconut milk)
   - Contains natural **medium-chain fats** that aid in better vitamin D absorption.

4. **Leafy Greens:** (like **spinach, kale, collard greens**)
   - Rich in **magnesium,** which is critical for activating vitamin D in the body.

5. **Mushrooms:** (especially sun-exposed mushrooms like **shiitake, maitake, portobello**)
   - Mushrooms themselves contain **vitamin D2,** and pairing them with healthy fats boosts absorption.

6. **Olives and Cold-Pressed Olive Oil:**
   - Excellent source of **monounsaturated fats** that aid in fat-soluble vitamin absorption naturally.

7. **Sweet Potatoes:**
   - High in **potassium** and **magnesium**, supporting overall vitamin D functions.

8. **Legumes:** (like **lentils, chickpeas, mung beans**)
   - Provide **magnesium and zinc**, minerals involved in vitamin D utilization.

9. **Tahini:** (Sesame Seed Paste)
   - Very rich in **healthy fats** and **minerals** like magnesium and zinc.

🌸 Important Tips for Natural Vitamin D Boost:
   - **Sunlight first:** Skin exposure to sunlight (morning sun) is your *best natural source.*
   - **Eat plant fats with sun-exposed foods:** For example, enjoy a **mushroom-avocado salad** after sunbathing!
   - **Stay hydrated:** Good hydration also helps the liver and kidneys, which activate vitamin D.

✦ Quick Healing Tip for Readers:

"Combine sun exposure with a magnesium-rich, plant-based meal to maximize your body's natural vitamin D activation."

2. 💧 The Power of Hydration – How Water Heals the Body

Water is essential for every cellular process: detoxification, digestion, circulation, and temperature regulation.

◇ Key Points:
   - Water makes up **60-70% of the body** and is essential for every cellular function.
   - Proper hydration **flushes toxins, improves digestion, and keeps joints lubricated.**
   - Chronic dehydration contributes to **fatigue, headaches, kidney stones, poor digestion and aging skin.**

- Structured water (spring water, mineral-rich water from raw fruits, vegetables, and coconut water) hydrates more effectively than tap or processed water.

◇ **Optimal Hydration Practices:**

- ✔ **Drink at least half your body weight in ounces** (e.g., 150 lbs = 75 oz daily).
- ✔ **Start the day with warm lemon water** to cleanse the digestive system.
- ✔ **Add sea salt or minerals** to water for better electrolyte balance.
- ✔ **Avoid plastic bottles;** use glass or stainless steel to prevent chemical exposure.

◇ **Examples & Interesting Facts:**

- **Mild dehydration can lower energy levels by 30%** and cause brain fog.
- **Drinking water before meals aids digestion and prevents overeating.**
- **Natural spring water is one of the richest sources of minerals,** crucial for health.
- Drinking water first thing in the morning flushes out toxins and jumpstarts metabolism.

◇ **Actionable Tip for Readers:**

- Try **herbal-infused water (mint, lemon, ginger) for enhanced hydration and detoxification.**
- Start your day with **warm lemon water or coconut water** to hydrate and alkalize your body.
- Include hydrating foods like cucumbers, watermelon, oranges, and celery in your meals.

3. 🌍 Grounding and Earthing: How Reconnecting with Nature Restores Balance

✿ What Is Earthing or Grounding?

Earthing, also known as **grounding**, is the practice of connecting your body directly with the Earth's surface—most commonly by walking barefoot on grass, soil, sand, or even unpainted concrete. It might sound simple, but this age-old practice holds **profound healing potential** backed by modern science and ancient wisdom.

Earthing involves making **skin contact with the Earth's natural surfaces,** allowing free electrons from the Earth to flow into your body. These electrons are powerful **antioxidants** that help neutralize free radicals in your body, reducing **inflammation, pain, and stress.**

💜 Health Benefits of Walking Barefoot on Grass

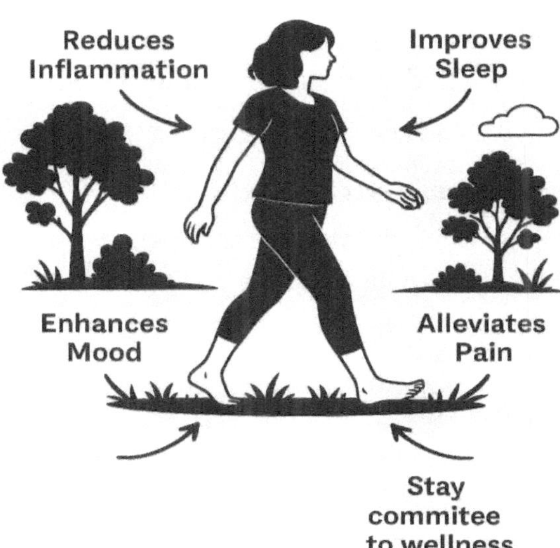

1. **Reduces Chronic Inflammation:**
   - Chronic inflammation is the root cause of many modern diseases—from arthritis to heart problems.
   - Earthing reduces markers of inflammation by balancing the body's electrical charge and calming the immune response.

2. **Improves Sleep and Energy:**
   - Walking barefoot helps reset your circadian rhythm.
   - It calms the nervous system, helping you fall asleep faster and wake up more refreshed.

3. **Pain Relief and Muscle Recovery:**
   - Studies show that earthing reduces **pain, muscle stiffness,** and **delayed-onset muscle soreness** (DOMS), especially in those with joint or nerve issues.

4. **Lowers Stress and Anxiety:**
   - Earthing helps reduce **cortisol levels,** leading to a calm, centered feeling—making it an excellent tool for mental health and emotional stability.

5. **Supports Heart Health:**
   - It improves blood viscosity and flow, which can help prevent **blood clots** and improve overall cardiovascular function.

6. **Balances the Autonomic Nervous System:**
   - Grounding supports the **parasympathetic (rest and digest)** nervous system, which promotes healing and reduces stress-related disease.

☺ Personal Experience:

In my own healing journey, **walking barefoot on grass every morning in the sunlight** became a sacred ritual. The warmth of the Earth beneath my feet and the serenity of nature helped me **release stress,** regain **mental clarity,** and ease **physical discomfort.** Over time, it became a powerful catalyst in my journey to reverse high blood pressure and boost emotional resilience—without medication.

✿ How to Practice Earthing:

- **Walk barefoot** for 20–30 minutes daily on natural surfaces like grass, sand, or soil.
- **Lie on the ground,** garden with bare hands, or sit with feet touching the Earth.
- Use **grounding mats or sheets** indoors if going outside is not always possible.

🌍 Final Thought:

"The Earth has energy meant to heal you—if only you pause, remove your shoes, and receive."

Earthing is simple, free, and incredibly powerful. When you reconnect with the Earth, you're not just healing your body—you're returning to a natural rhythm that's been waiting for you all along.

◇ Key Points:

- **Walking barefoot on natural surfaces (grass, sand, soil) allows the body to absorb Earth's electrons,** reducing inflammation, stress and improves sleep.
- The modern lifestyle (rubber-soled shoes, concrete buildings) **disconnects us from the Earth's healing energy.**
- Scientific studies show **Grounding lowers cortisol, improves sleep, and reduces chronic pain.**It helps balance the nervous system and reduces stress by restoring the body's natural electrical state.

◇ Ways to Practice Grounding:

- ✔ Walk barefoot outside for at least 10-20 minutes daily.
- ✔ **Lie on the grass or beach** to maximize skin-to-earth contact.

- ✔ **Use grounding mats or sheets indoors** if outdoor access is limited.
- ✔ **Practice gardening**—handling soil has been shown to improve mood (due to beneficial microbes).

◇ **Examples & Interesting Facts:**

- **A 2012 study found grounding can reduce blood viscosity,** lowering the risk of heart disease.
- **Earthing therapy has been shown to speed up wound healing.**
- **Hugging a tree or sitting under it** can have calming effects due to phytoncides (natural compounds trees release).
- Research shows that grounding can **reduce blood viscosity, a** major factor in cardiovascular disease.

◇ **Actionable Tip for Readers:**

- Take **a 15-minute barefoot walk in the grass each morning** to reset your nervous system.
- Make "earthing" a part of your morning ritual—go barefoot on the grass while soaking in the sunlight. Double the healing benefits!

Example: A daily practice of **walking barefoot for 30–45 minutes** on grass helped Reena experience emotional calm, lower blood pressure, and a deeper sense of connection to the Earth.

4. ⌂ Forest Bathing, Fresh Air, and Natural Environments for Stress Reduction

Nature exposure reduces cortisol levels, lowers heart rate, and boosts mood and immunity.

◇ **Key Points:**

- Spending time in forests or natural spaces **lowers stress hormones, enhances immune function, and improves mental clarity.**

- Trees release **phytoncides, natural compounds that boost immune cells (NK cells).**
- Exposure to fresh air increases **oxygen levels in the blood, improving brain function and mood.**
- Natural environments activate the parasympathetic nervous system—your body's rest-and-heal mode.

◇ **How to Reap the Benefits:**
- ✔ **Practice Shinrin-Yoku (Japanese forest bathing)**—walk slowly, breathe deeply, and immerse in nature.
- ✔ **Take breaks outdoors** instead of staying in artificial environments all day.
- ✔ **Go hiking, sit by a river, or listen to birds**—natural sounds are scientifically proven to lower stress.

◇ **Examples & Interesting Facts:**
- **A study in Japan found that forest bathing reduces cortisol by 16% and blood pressure by 2%.**
- **People who live near green spaces have lower rates of anxiety and depression.**
- **Breathing in ocean air (rich in negative ions) enhances lung function and serotonin production.**
- Trees release **phytoncides,** antimicrobial compounds that boost natural killer (NK) cell activity in the immune system.

◇ **Actionable Tip for Readers:**
- Spend **30 minutes in nature weekly** to reduce stress and boost immunity.
- Plan weekly nature escapes—visit parks, gardens, or nature trails. Even **5 minutes of fresh air and sunlight** on your balcony can uplift your spirit.

Example: Spending just **20 minutes in a natural environment** can lower stress hormones and elevate mood significantly.

Conclusion of the Chapter

☑ Summarize the key ideas:

- Sunlight fuels Vitamin D production, boosts mood, and strengthens immunity.
- Hydration is essential for detoxification, energy, and brain function.
- Grounding connects the body to the Earth's healing energy, reducing inflammation.
- Spending time in nature relieves stress, strengthens immunity, and enhances well-being.

◇ **Final Takeaway for Readers:**

- Make **sunlight, water, grounding and nature** a daily habit to experience profound health benefits.

7-Day Nature Healing Challenge

This challenge will help readers integrate **sunlight, water, and grounding** into their daily routines for **better energy, reduced stress, and overall well-being.** Each day focuses on **one core natural healing practice,** building momentum for lifelong habits.

Day 1: Morning Sunlight & Deep Breathing ☼ ❁

Goal: Reset your circadian rhythm, boost mood, and energize your body.

☑ Spend **10-20 minutes in morning sunlight** (before 10 AM) without sunglasses.

☑ Practice **deep breathing** (inhale for 4 sec, hold for 4 sec, exhale for 6 sec) for relaxation.

☑ Bonus: Take a **short walk outdoors** while soaking up the sun.

◇ **Why it Works:** Morning light regulates **melatonin and serotonin,** improving sleep and mood.

Day 2: Hydration & Detox Water 💧 🜕

Goal: Flush toxins, boost digestion, and rehydrate cells.

- ☑ Start the day with **a glass of warm lemon water.**
- ☑ Drink **at least 8-10 glasses of filtered/mineral-rich water.**
- ☑ Bonus: Try **herbal-infused water** (mint, ginger, cucumber) for extra detox benefits.

  ◇ **Why it Works:** Hydration supports **cellular repair, brain function, and energy levels.**

Day 3: Barefoot Grounding & Nature Connection 🌐 👣

Goal: Absorb Earth's natural energy to reduce stress and inflammation.

- ☑ Walk **barefoot on grass, soil, or sand** for at least **15 minutes.**
- ☑ If barefoot isn't possible, **sit outside with hands or feet touching the earth.**
- ☑ Bonus: Try **gardening, hugging a tree, or meditating outdoors.**

  ◇ **Why it Works:** Grounding balances **electrical charges in the body,** reducing stress and improving sleep.

Day 4: Forest Bathing & Natural Air Therapy 🜄 🌿

Goal: Lower stress and increase oxygen levels by immersing in nature.

- ☑ Spend at least **30 minutes in a park, forest, or by water.**
- ☑ Engage all senses: **Touch leaves, listen to birds, smell fresh air, and feel the breeze.**
- ☑ Bonus: Practice **Shinrin-Yoku (Japanese forest bathing)**—walk slowly and mindfully.

  ◇ **Why it Works:** Forest air releases **phytoncides,** which boost immune cells and reduce cortisol.

Day 5: Sun Therapy & Vitamin D Boost ○ ✐

Goal: Improve Vitamin D levels and strengthen immunity.

- ☑ Expose **arms, legs, or back to direct sunlight for 15-30 minutes** (without sunscreen).
- ☑ If sunlight is limited, eat **Vitamin D-rich foods** (orange juice,soaked almonds and seeds,mushrooms, chia seeds and flax seeds.
- ☑ Bonus: Take **a short midday sun break** for added energy.

◇ **Why it Works:** Vitamin D is essential for **bone health, mood stability, and disease prevention.**

Day 6: Water Immersion & Cold Therapy 🫧 ❄

Goal: Improve circulation, reduce pain, and boost energy.

- ☑ Take a **cold shower or splash cold water** on your face in the morning.
- ☑ If possible, **immerse in natural water** (ocean, lake, river) for a few minutes.
- ☑ Bonus: Alternate between **warm and cold water** to increase blood flow.

◇ **Why it Works:** Cold water **reduces inflammation, strengthens the nervous system, and improves focus.**

Day 7: Mindful Nature Ritual & Reflection ❀ 🧘

Goal: Create a lifelong connection with nature for healing and peace.

- ☑ Spend **quiet time in nature**—meditate, stretch, or sit mindfully.
- ☑ Reflect on how the **past 6 days have improved your well-being.**
- ☑ Bonus: Journal about **how you'll continue incorporating nature into your daily life.**

◇ **Why it Works:** Nature therapy **lowers stress, improves creativity, and enhances emotional resilience.**

Final Takeaway for Readers

❇ This challenge is just the beginning—keep integrating **sunlight, water, and grounding** into your lifestyle for **lifelong health and vitality.**

☺ **Even small changes**—like drinking more water, walking barefoot on wet grass, or spending time in sunlight—**can have profound healing effects.**

🌀 **Reconnect with nature daily,** and your body will thank you.

Chapter 8

HOLISTIC THERAPIES FOR PAIN RELIEF AND LONGTIVITY

This chapter explores **ancient and modern holistic therapies** that support **natural healing, pain relief, and overall well-being.** These methods harness the body's **energy systems, touch, and sound frequencies** to restore balance and vitality.

✦ Motivational Quote

"Sometimes the most powerful healing doesn't come from medicine, but from hands that care, sounds that soothe, and energies that align."- Reena Agarwal

This quote will set the tone for you to explore the deep, nurturing wisdom of holistic touch and energy-based healing.

❀ My Healing Journey with Holistic Therapies

By Reena Agarwal

I vividly remember the time when my body was constantly aching. Long hours, poor posture, emotional stress—it all built up silently. Despite taking medications, the pain never truly went away. That's when I turned to holistic therapies, and everything began to change.

Every evening, I began dipping my legs in warm water infused with Epsom salt and essential oils. This simple act melted away fatigue and pain. I started receiving gentle reflexology sessions weekly, and I couldn't believe the difference. Pressure on my feet somehow relieved my stiff neck. It felt like my body was being reset.

Later, I discovered **Reiki**. Initially skeptical, I allowed myself to receive. The calm I felt during and after the session was unlike anything before—like being held in a gentle cocoon of light and warmth. I knew then that healing could happen even without touch, through intention and energy.

What began as an experiment became a way of life. Now, I integrate these therapies into my routine—Reiki for emotional clarity, sound healing before sleep, and self-massage with warm oils every weekend.

These aren't just therapies—they're rituals of love for my body and soul. And I truly believe they've helped me stay pain-free, peaceful, and radiant—without relying on medicine.

1. Acupressure, Massage, and Reflexology for Self-Healing

◇ **Key Points:**

These ancient touch-based therapies stimulate the body's innate healing mechanisms by activating pressure points, improving circulation, and balancing energy flow.

- **Acupressure** applies pressure to specific body points to **relieve pain, improve circulation, and balance energy flow.**
- **Massage therapy** helps **release muscle tension, reduce stress hormones, and improve lymphatic drainage.**
- **Reflexology** stimulates pressure points on the hands, feet, and ears to **promote organ function and reduce stress.**

◇ **How to Practice:**

- ✔ **Acupressure for headaches:** Press the LI4 (**Hegu**) point—between the thumb and index finger—for relief.
- ✔ **Self-massage:** Use circular motions on the neck, shoulders, and lower back to release tension.
- ✔ **Reflexology for better sleep:** Massage the **solar plexus point** (center of the foot) for relaxation.

◇ **Examples & Interesting Facts:**

- **A Harvard study found that massage therapy reduces cortisol levels by 31%** and boosts serotonin by 28%.

- A person suffering from chronic migraines may find relief through foot reflexology targeting the head and neck zones, combined with regular neck massages.

- **Acupressure has been used in Traditional Chinese Medicine for over 2,000 years** to unblock energy meridians.

- **Reflexology was practiced in Ancient Egypt**—pictographs of foot massage were found in tombs dating back to 2,500 BC.

◇ **Actionable Tip for Readers:**

- Try a **5-minute acupressure session daily** on tension points (head, hands, or feet) for stress relief

- Try a simple self-acupressure technique: apply firm pressure to the web between your thumb and index finger (LI-4 point) to relieve headaches and stress.

2. Sound Healing and Vibration Therapy

◇ **Key Points:**

Everything in the body is energy, including sound. Sound healing uses vibrations to bring the body's frequencies into harmony, reducing stress and restoring cellular balance.

- Sound frequencies affect the body at a **cellular level, helping to reduce stress and improve energy flow.**

- **Tuning forks, singing bowls, and binaural beats** create healing vibrations that resonate with the body's natural frequencies.

- Certain frequencies (e.g., **528 Hz for DNA repair, 432 Hz for relaxation**) promote healing and calm the nervous system

- ◇ **Ways to Experience Sound Healing:**
  - ✔ **Listen to Solfeggio frequencies** (528 Hz, 432 Hz, 639 Hz) for relaxation and cellular healing.
  - ✔ **Use Tibetan singing bowls or tuning forks** to rebalance energy and relieve pain.
  - ✔ **Chanting 'Om' or humming** creates vibrations that calm the nervous system.

- ◇ **Examples & Interesting Facts:**
  - NASA research shows that every organ and cell in the body has its own frequency—disease occurs when it's out of harmony.
  - Monks use sound therapy in meditation to shift brain waves into a healing state.
  - A 2016 study found that singing bowl therapy significantly reduces blood pressure and stress.
  - Regular exposure to singing bowl meditations has been shown to reduce anxiety and enhance deep sleep, especially in people with chronic stress.

- ◇ **Actionable Tip for Readers:**
  - Try **5 minutes of sound therapy** before bed—listen to **healing frequencies or use a singing bowl** for relaxation.
  - Start your day with 5 minutes of humming or listening to calming binaural beats to raise your vibrational frequency and support mental clarity.

3. The Role of Energy Medicine—Reiki, Acupuncture, and Biofeedback

- ◇ **Key Points:**

Energy medicine works with the body's electromagnetic field and energy pathways (chakras and meridians) to promote balance, remove blockages, and speed up healing.

- **Reiki** is a Japanese technique that uses **gentle touch to transfer healing energy** and balance the body's chakras.

- **Acupuncture** (inserting fine needles into energy meridians) helps **relieve pain, improve circulation, and restore organ function.**

- **Biofeedback** measures physiological responses (heart rate, brain waves, muscle tension) to help people **control stress and pain consciously.**

◇ **How to Experience Energy Healing:**

✔ **Try a Reiki session** for deep relaxation and emotional healing.

✔ **Acupressure (DIY acupuncture):** Stimulate meridian points by applying firm pressure.

✔ **Use biofeedback apps or wearable devices** to monitor and control stress responses.

◇ **Examples & Interesting Facts:**

- **Reiki has been used in over 800 hospitals worldwide** to support patient recovery.

- **Acupuncture is scientifically proven to release endorphins,** reducing pain and inflammation.

- **The U.S. military has incorporated biofeedback into stress management programs for soldiers.**

- A woman with chronic back pain experiences more relief through regular Reiki and acupuncture than from years of painkillers.

◇ **Actionable Tip for Readers:**

- Try a **simple Reiki self-healing practice:**. Place one hand over your heart and the other on your solar plexus (just above the navel) for 10 minutes daily to soothe anxiety and tension, take deep breaths, and visualize warm energy flowing through your body.

4. Healing Touch: The Power of Human Connection and Positive Energy

◇ **Key Points:**

Physical touch and emotional connection play a vital role in healing. Touch stimulates oxytocin release, reduces cortisol, and enhances overall well-being.

Healing touch isn't only physical—it's about **presence, intention,** and **energy exchange.** A caring hug, holding hands, or a loving gaze can spark physiological healing responses.

- Human touch **releases oxytocin, lowers stress hormones, and boosts the immune system.**

- **Therapeutic touch (TT) and emotional support from others** can enhance recovery from illness and surgery.

- **Loving-kindness meditation** (sending positive energy to oneself and others) **creates emotional and physical healing effects.**

◇ **Ways to Use Healing Touch:**

- ✔ Hug therapy: Aim for **at least 8 hugs a day** for emotional well-being.

- ✔ Practice self-touch: Place a hand on your heart or stomach to activate relaxation responses.

- ✔ Hold hands or gently massage loved ones—even simple touch reduces stress and improves emotional connection.

◇ **Examples & Interesting Facts:**

- Studies show that premature babies who receive skin-to-skin contact gain weight faster and have stronger immune systems.

- Therapeutic touch is now being integrated into palliative care for chronic pain relief.

- A hug lasting 20 seconds releases oxytocin, reducing cortisol and lowering blood pressure.

- Studies have shown that premature babies gain weight faster and experience better development when given daily skin-to-skin contact.

- People living alone with chronic conditions often improve when regularly receiving therapeutic touch or simply being surrounded by positive, supportive energy.

◇ **Actionable Tip for Readers:**
  - Try **a 30-second self-hug or a hand massage** to activate relaxation and energy flow.
  - Practice **"mindful touch"** with a loved one—place your hand on their shoulder with intention, compassion, and presence. Notice how both of you feel grounded and comforted.

Conclusion of the Chapter

☑ Summarize the key ideas:
  - **Acupressure, massage, and reflexology** offer drug-free pain relief and relaxation.
  - **Sound healing and vibration therapy** realign the body's energy for emotional and physical well-being.
  - **Energy medicine (Reiki, acupuncture, biofeedback)** restores balance and promotes healing.
  - **Human touch and positive energy** strengthen immunity, reduce pain, and enhance mental health.

◇ **Final Takeaway for Readers:**
  - **Integrate one holistic therapy into your routine**—whether it's self-massage, sound healing, or grounding touch—to experience profound benefits.

✦ Summary:

These therapies are not just alternatives—they are ancient and evidence-backed ways to **restore balance, relieve pain,** and promote **longevity.** They remind us that healing isn't always in a pill—sometimes, it's in a soft touch, a gentle sound, or a silent intention.

Chapter 9

CREATING A SUSTAINABLE, DISEASE-FREE LIFESTYLE

"Wellness is not a destination—it is a daily journey of mindful choices. Each simple habit is a step toward a vibrant, disease-free life."

❄ This chapter will help readers **turn natural healing principles into a long-term lifestyle** by creating **daily habits, adapting to different life stages, and overcoming challenges.** The focus is on **practical strategies** for **lifelong health, vitality, and resilience.**

1. How to Build Lifelong Habits That Prevent Illness

◇ **Key Points:**

Creating a healthy lifestyle isn't about short bursts of change—it's about building habits that last. The key is **consistency over perfection.**

- **Prevention is better than cure**—building small, consistent habits reduces the risk of chronic diseases.

- **Start small and build gradually:** Begin with a daily morning detox drink, then add in yoga or meditation.

- **Make it enjoyable:** Choose natural healing practices that resonate with you—whether it's herbal teas, barefoot walks, or journaling.

- **Pair habits with existing routines:** Do deep breathing while waiting for tea to brew or stretch while watching TV.

- **The power of micro-changes**: Small daily choices **compound over time** into lasting health benefits.
- **Identify and eliminate triggers** that lead to unhealthy choices (processed foods, sedentary lifestyle, chronic stress).

◇ **Examples & Interesting Facts:**

- **Studies show that 80% of chronic diseases (heart disease, diabetes, obesity) are preventable with lifestyle changes.**
- **The Okinawans (Japan) live the longest because of simple habits:** a whole-food diet, regular movement, purpose-driven living, and strong social connections.
- **A Harvard study found that people who maintain 5 key habits (healthy diet, exercise, no smoking, moderate alcohol, and weight management) live 10+ years longer.**

Reena begins each morning with a glass of warm lemon water, followed by yoga and barefoot grounding. This became her non-negotiable foundation for the day—simple, yet transformative.

Actionable Tips for Readers:

✔ Use **habit stacking** (e.g., drink water before brushing teeth) to make health habits automatic.

✔ Keep a **daily wellness tracker** for consistency (sunlight, hydration, movement, mindfulness).

✔ Follow the **80/20 rule**—prioritize nutrient-rich, healing foods 80% of the time but allow flexibility.

💡 **Actionable Tip:**

Choose **one habit** to commit to for the next 21 days. Track it on a calendar and reward yourself for consistency.

2. Daily Routines for Optimal Health and Vitality

◇ **Key Points:**

Your daily routine is your medicine. By creating rituals aligned with natural rhythms, you support your body's healing systems effortlessly.

◇ **Morning Rituals:**

- Warm lemon water or herbal detox drink
- Barefoot walk on grass (grounding)
- 20–45 minutes of yoga and deep breathing
- Light fruit-based breakfast or green juice

◇ **Afternoon Boost:**

- Hydrate regularly with copper or clay pot water
- Light lunch of sprouts, raw salads, and healthy fats
- Short rest or silent time (if possible)

◇ **Evening Calm:**

- Soothing herbal tea (e.g., tulsi or chamomile)
- Warm foot soak or oil massage
- Gratitude journaling or meditation

◇ **Key Ideas:**

A structured **morning, afternoon, and evening wellness routine** helps maintain balance.

- **Morning rituals set the tone for the day** (hydration, movement, sunlight exposure).
- **Midday energy boosters** (breathwork, grounding, mindful eating) sustain energy.
- **Evening wind-down routines** (herbal teas, no screens, gratitude practice) improve sleep quality.

◇ **Ideal Daily Wellness Routine:**

☺ **Morning:**

- ✔ **Drink 1-2 glasses of water** to flush toxins.
- ✔ **Get 10-20 minutes of sunlight** to regulate circadian rhythms.
- ✔ **Move your body** (yoga, stretching, or a walk).

❋ **Midday:**

- ✔ **Eat a nutrient-dense meal** with anti-inflammatory foods.
- ✔ **Breathe deeply or take a short nature break** to reset energy.
- ✔ **Practice gratitude or a mindful pause** to reduce stress.

☾ **Evening:**

- ✔ **Unplug from screens** at least 1 hour before bed.
- ✔ **Drink a calming herbal tea** (chamomile, ashwagandha, or valerian root).
- ✔ **Practice a sleep ritual** (journaling, deep breathing, light stretching).

◇ **Interesting Facts:**

- • **Research shows** that people who follow a structured morning routine have lower stress levels and higher productivity.
- • **Taking a 10-minute nature break** mid-day can improve focus and reduce cortisol levels.
- • **Blue light from screens** disrupts melatonin production, reducing sleep quality by up to 50%.

✍ **Example:** One of Reena's most powerful habits was creating a "no-gadget zone" after 8 PM—leading to deeper sleep and more emotional balance.

◇ **Actionable Tip for Readers:**

Create a personalized daily wellness routine that incorporates one small habit at a time.

💡 **Actionable Tip:**

Craft your own *healing daily rhythm*—a simple 3-step morning and evening practice that you can sustain.

3. Adapting Natural Healing to Different Life Stages

Whether you're in your 20s or 70s, natural healing can be tailored to fit your life stage.

◇ **For Young Adults (20s–30s):**
- Focus on energy, skin, and immunity.
- Incorporate raw foods, juices, grounding, and mental clarity through meditation.

◇ **For Middle Age (40s–60s):**
- Prioritize hormonal balance, stress reduction, and joint flexibility.
- Include more anti-inflammatory foods, yoga, and mindful relaxation.

◇ **For Seniors (60+):**
- Focus on bone strength, digestion, and calmness.
- Gentle stretching, sun exposure, warm soups, and nature walks are key.

◇ **Key Points:**
- **Wellness looks different at every age**—each life stage has specific nutritional and lifestyle needs.
- **Teens & Young Adults:** Focus on **hormonal balance, brain health, and stress management.**
- **30s-40s:** Prioritize **gut health, metabolism, and energy optimization.**
- **50s-60s+:** Strengthen **bones, heart, and cognitive function with anti-aging strategies.**

- ◇ **Tailored Health Strategies by Age:**
  - ✔ **20s-30s:** Build **strong habits early**—focus on whole foods, fitness, and emotional resilience.
  - ✔ **40s-50s:** Support **hormonal changes** with adaptogenic herbs (maca, ashwagandha).
  - ✔ **60s+:** Protect **cognitive and joint health** with omega-3s, turmeric, and daily movement.

- ◇ **Interesting Facts:**
  - • Natural plant diet followers in their 50s have a 40% lower risk of developing dementia later in life.
  - • Strength training twice a week after 40 helps prevent osteoporosis and age-related muscle loss.
  - • People who maintain social connections as they age have a 50% higher chance of living longer.

📌 **Example:** Reena introduced her 70-year-old aunt to daily **sunbathing and lemon ginger tea.** Within months, her energy and digestion significantly improved.

- ◇ **Actionable Tip for Readers:**
  - • **Create an age-specific health checklist** to ensure optimal well-being at every stage of life.

💡 **Actionable Tip:**

Every few years, reassess your **natural healing practices** and gently update your routine to fit your body's evolving needs.

4. Overcoming Obstacles and Staying Committed to Wellness

- ◇ **Key Points:**

Even the best intentions can be challenged by time constraints, social situations, or emotional dips. What matters is **getting back on track—without guilt.**

◇ **Common Obstacles:**

- **Identify common barriers:** lack of time, motivation, support or conflicting health information.
- **Create accountability**—join wellness groups, find a health buddy, or track progress.
- **Develop a flexible mindset**—wellness is not about perfection but **progress and consistency.**
- **Temptation** for old food habits
- **Emotional eating** or stress triggers

◇ **Solutions:**

- Create a supportive environment—clear your kitchen of junk, join like-minded wellness groups.
- Prepare and plan meals ahead.
- Reframe "cheat days" as "choice days"—and enjoy mindfully.

◇ **Ways to Stay on Track:**

- ✔ Set small, achievable goals instead of overwhelming resolutions.
- ✔ **Surround yourself with positive influences** (supportive friends, books, podcasts).
- ✔ **Reframe setbacks as learning opportunities**—adjust and keep moving forward.

◇ **Interesting Facts:**

- **People who track their habits are 42% more likely to maintain long-term success.**
- **Community support increases the likelihood of achieving health goals by up to 95%.**
- **It takes an average of 66 days to form a new habit**—consistency is key.

⊁ **Example:** Reena often faced cravings for snacks during family gatherings. Instead of resisting, she brought her own date-nut laddoos and herbal drinks. Gradually, others joined her!

◇ **Actionable Tip for Readers:**

- Write down **3 wellness habits** you want to commit to for the next 30 days.

♀ **Actionable Tip:**

Create a **Wellness Emergency Kit**—including healthy snacks, herbal teas, uplifting quotes, and calming essential oils. Use it when life throws you off balance.

Conclusion of the Chapter

☑ Summarize the key ideas:

- **Lifelong wellness starts with small, daily habits**—focus on **hydration, movement, mindset, and nutrition.**
- **A structured daily routine** (morning, midday, evening) creates consistency.
- **Adapt natural healing practices** to different life stages for optimal health.
- **Overcoming obstacles and staying committed** ensures long-term well-being.

◇ **Final Takeaway for Readers:**

- True health isn't about quick fixes—it's about small, consistent choices that create a disease-free, vibrant life.

✿ Closing Message for the Chapter

Building a disease-free life is not about deprivation—it's about **living in harmony with nature and yourself.** Let your routine become your healing prayer. Let your lifestyle reflect self-love.

♀ *"A timeless guide to restoring health and vitality through the wisdom of nature."*

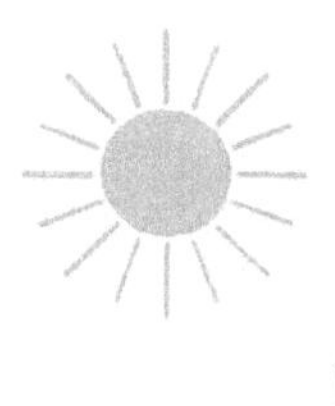

My Healing Daily Routine

'Let your daily rituals become the rhythm of your healing and the whispers of self-care.'

Morning

Afternoon

Evening

Conclusion

YOUR JOURNEY TO AGELESS HEALING BEGINS NOW

The conclusion should **empower you** to take action and integrate natural healing into their daily lives. It should leave them **inspired, confident, and motivated** to embrace a lifelong path of **vitality, balance, and wellness** without dependency on medication.

1. Recap of the Key Principles

◇ **Summarize the core lessons** from the book to reinforce their importance:

🌱 **Your body is designed to heal itself** when given the right nourishment, movement, and mindset.

- 🍏 **Food is medicine**—choosing whole, plant-based, and anti-inflammatory foods promotes healing.

- 🏃 **Daily movement and breathwork** improve circulation, reduce stress, and enhance longevity.

- 🧘 **Mind-body connection is powerful**—meditation, mindfulness, and stress reduction are essential for well-being.

- 🌿 **Nature's remedies (herbs, sunlight, grounding, water therapy)** are powerful tools for healing.

- 💚 **Holistic therapies (massage, acupressure, energy healing, etc.)** can naturally relieve pain and restore balance.

- 🕐 **True healing is a lifelong journey**—small, consistent habits create lasting health.

◇ **Example:**

"**By applying these principles,** you're not just preventing disease—you're unlocking the secret to a vibrant, thriving life at any age."

◇ **Actionable Tip:**

Encourage readers to reflect: What resonated with them the most? Which healing habits do they feel excited to start?

2. A 30-Day Action Plan for Implementing Natural Healing

Given a simple, step-by-step plan to apply what you have learned. **Each week focuses on a specific area,** making the transition manageable.

Week 1: Nutrition & Hydration

- ☑ Replace processed foods with whole, natural ingredients.
- ☑ Drink **at least 8 glasses of water daily** for detoxification.
- ☑ Start the day with a **healing herbal tea (ginger, turmeric, or green tea).**

Week 2: Movement & Breathwork

- ☑ Walk **at least 20 minutes daily** to improve circulation.
- ☑ Try **gentle yoga or stretching** in the morning or before bed.
- ☑ Practice **deep belly breathing (4-7-8 method) to lower stress.**

Week 3: Mind-Body Connection & Stress Reduction

- ☑ Meditate for **5-10 minutes daily** to enhance clarity and inner peace.
- ☑ Create a **sleep ritual**—dim lights, avoid screens, and relax before bed.
- ☑ Keep a **gratitude journal** to shift your mindset toward positivity.

Week 4: Nature & Holistic Healing

- ☑ Spend **10-15 minutes in sunlight** for vitamin D and energy.
- ☑ Try grounding—**walk barefoot on grass or soil** for balance.
- ☑ Use a **natural remedy (herbs, essential oils, or acupressure)** for a minor ailment.

◇ **Encouraging Note:**

"This is not a challenge—it's an invitation to start living in alignment with nature. Choose what works best for you and adapt as needed."

3. Encouragement and Motivation to Embrace a Thriving, Medicine-Free Life

💡 **Key Messages:**

- **Healing is a personal journey**—everyone moves at their own pace.
- **Progress over perfection**—even small changes can bring profound benefits.
- **Trust your body's wisdom**—it was designed to thrive naturally.
- **You are in control of your health**—every choice you make matters.

✴ **Inspiring Call to Action:**

- "Imagine waking up every morning feeling **energized, pain-free, and vibrant**—this is possible when you commit to natural healing."
- "The best time to start was yesterday. The second-best time is now."
- "You hold the power to heal, thrive, and live a life free from unnecessary medication. **Nature has always had the answers—now, it's time to embrace them.**"

Final Takeaway:

I encourage you to **continue your journey** by:

- ☑ Revisiting the book whenever you need inspiration.
- ☑ Sharing your healing journey with friends or family.
- ☑ Exploring deeper into holistic health through further reading and practice.

Here are some **journal prompts** and a **printable habit tracker** idea to help you stay committed to their healing journey.

📖 Journal Prompts for Reflection & Healing

Encourage readers to **journal daily or weekly** to track their progress, uncover patterns, and stay motivated.

1. **Self-Discovery & Healing Intentions:**
   - What does "ageless healing" mean to me?
   - What are my top three health goals for the next six months?
   - How do I currently feel in my body, mind, and spirit? What do I want to improve?
   - What small step can I take today to prioritize my health naturally?

2. **Nutrition & Nourishment:**
   - How does my body feel after eating whole, natural foods versus processed foods?
   - Which foods make me feel energized and which ones make me sluggish?
   - What is one new healing food or herb I want to incorporate this week?

3. **Movement & Breathwork:**
   - How does my mood shift after moving my body?
   - Which form of exercise or movement feels best for me right now?
   - How do I feel after practicing deep breathing for a few minutes?

4. **Stress, Sleep & Emotional Well-being:**
   - What is currently causing me stress, and how can I release it?
   - What nighttime ritual can I implement to improve my sleep?
   - What am I grateful for today?

5. Connecting with Nature & Holistic Healing:

- How do I feel after spending time outdoors?
- What natural remedy (herb, essential oil, acupressure, etc.) has helped me the most?
- How can I make nature a bigger part of my daily routine?

📋 Printable Habit Tracker for a 30-Day Healing Plan

A **visual habit tracker** can help readers stay on track with small, daily healing habits.

❀ Categories to Track Daily:

- ☑ Hydration (8+ glasses of water)
- ☑ Eating whole, plant-rich foods
- ☑ 15-30 minutes of movement
- ☑ Deep breathing or meditation
- ☑ 10+ minutes in sunlight/nature
- ☑ Practicing gratitude or journaling
- ☑ Using a natural remedy (herb, essential oil, acupressure, etc.)

🗓 **Readers can mark off each habit daily and track progress over time.**

Habit Tracker

Ageless Healing Through Nature: 30-Day Habit Tracker

How to Use This Tracker:

- Each day, check off the habits you complete.
- Aim for consistency, not perfection. Even small steps lead to big results.
- Reflect at the end of the month on what worked best for you.

Daily Healing Habits Checklist

Day	Hydration (8+ glasses)	Whole Foods & Healing Nutrition	15+ min Movement	Deep Breathing / Meditation	10+ min Sunlight/Nature	Gratitude / Journaling	Natural Remedy (Herbs, Essential Oils, etc.)
1							
2							
3							
4							
5							
6							
7							
8							
9							
10							

Day	Hydration (8+ glasses)	Whole Foods & Healing Nutrition	15+ min Movement	Deep Breathing / Meditation	10+ min Sunlight/Nature	Gratitude / Journaling	Natural Remedy (Herbs, Essential Oils, etc.)
11							
12							
13							
14							
15							
16							
17							
18							
19							
20							

Day	Hydration (8+ glasses)	Whole Foods & Healing Nutrition	15+ min Movement	Deep Breathing / Meditation	10+ min Sunlight/Nature	Gratitude / Journaling	Natural Remedy (Herbs, Essential Oils, etc.)
21							
22							
23							
24							
25							
26							
27							
28							
29							
30							

End of Month Reflection Questions

1. Which habit was the easiest for me to maintain? Why?
2. Which habit was the most challenging? How can I make it easier?
3. What positive changes did I notice in my body, mind, or energy levels?
4. How do I feel about my progress, and what will I continue next month?

✦ **Remember:** Healing is a journey, not a race. Every step you take brings you closer to a vibrant, medicine-free life! Keep going! ❀ ♡

I've created a **30-day habit tracker** with a daily checklist and reflection questions to help you stay on track.

BONUS SECTION

Quick-Reference Healing Guide for Common Ailments

A simple, easy-to-use guide that lists natural remedies for common health concerns. Includes:

- **Headaches & Migraines** – Herbal teas (peppermint, ginger), acupressure points, and hydration tips.

- **Digestive Issues** – Soaked fennel seeds, probiotic-rich foods, and mindful eating practices.

- **Joint Pain & Inflammation** – Turmeric and black pepper, Epsom salt baths, gentle yoga.

- **Sleep Troubles & Stress** – Magnesium-rich foods, guided meditation, lavender essential oil.

- **Immune Support** – Raw honey, vitamin C-rich fruits, and deep breathing exercises.

Simple Meal Plans and Recipes for Natural Healing

A 7-day meal plan with easy-to-follow recipes that support healing and overall wellness. Featuring:

- **Breakfast:** Fresh fruit bowls with soaked seeds and nuts, fresh fruits and vegetable juices, green smoothies, herbal teas.

- **Lunch:** Nourishing salads with sprouts, avocado, and a variety of colorful vegetables.

- **Dinner:** Light, plant-based soups, steamed greens, and wholesome grains like quinoa or millet.

- **Snacks:** Coconut water, fresh coconut, homemade energy balls, and soaked dry fruits.

- **Healing Drinks:** Turmeric golden milk of dry fruits (dairy-free), detox herbal teas, and rejuvenating fresh juices.

This bonus section serves as a practical toolkit to help readers integrate natural healing into their daily lives effortlessly.

Disclaimer

Please note: All content shared here is based on my personal journey and professional experience. While the approaches described have been effective for me and many others, individual results may vary. If you have any existing medical conditions or concerns, I encourage you to consult your healthcare provider before making any major lifestyle changes. The author cannot take responsibility for any complications arising from the misuse of the information in this book.

Thank You for Joining This Healing Journey! ❧

If *Ageless Healing Through Nature* has touched your life, inspired positive changes, or simply given you hope — I would be deeply grateful if you could take a moment to leave a review on the site where you purchased this book.

Your words not only encourage me but also help others discover a natural path to wellness and vitality.

I'd also love to hear your personal healing stories or reflections!

Feel free to write to me at **reenaagarwal1964@gmail.com** — your journey matters, and together, we can inspire many more to choose healing through nature. ✿

With heartfelt gratitude,

– Reena Agarwal